Dear Paul,

With Best Wishes

from Isam Mochizuki

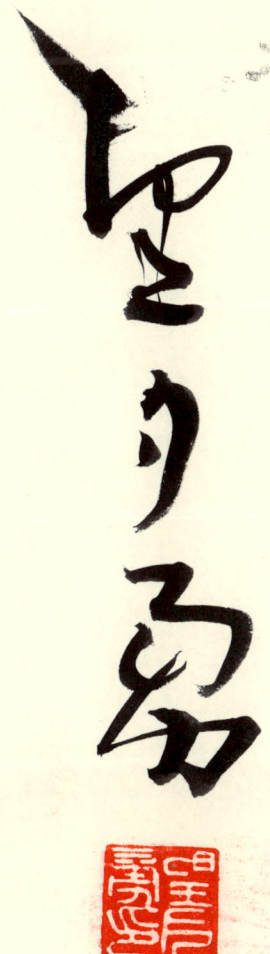

The Power Of Life

by

Mr. Isamu Mochizuki

Translated by Simon Grisdale

Bloomington, IN authorHOUSE® Milton Keynes, UK

AuthorHouse™
1663 Liberty Drive, Suite 200
Bloomington, IN 47403
www.authorhouse.com
Phone: 1-800-839-8640

AuthorHouse™ UK Ltd.
500 Avebury Boulevard
Central Milton Keynes, MK9 2BE
www.authorhouse.co.uk
Phone: 08001974150

© *2007 Mr. Isamu Mochizuki. All rights reserved.*

No part of this book may be reproduced, stored in a retrieval system, or transmitted by any means without the written permission of the author.

First published by AuthorHouse 2/20/2007

ISBN: 978-1-4259-6318-7 (sc)
ISBN: 978-1-4259-6319-4 (hc)

Printed in the United States of America
Bloomington, Indiana

This book is printed on acid-free paper.

The original Japanese version of The Power of Life "Inochinochikara" was published by Heibonsha Publishers, Tokyo, on 25th November 2004.

Table of Contents

The Translator xi

Chapter 1: The Journey Of Life 1
   The Meaning Of Being 'Allowed' To Live 3
   My Experiences After I Stopped Thinking Negatively 4
   Relying On Intuition 6
   Getting Rid Of An Attachment To Things 8
   A Stirring Image In An Ancient Hindi Temple 9
   A Wonderful Experience Of Becoming One With Nature 10
   Stung By A Scorpion And Thinking Of Home 12
   In The Desert, Knowledge Becomes Wisdom 14
   Life Revolves Like A Wheel 16

Chapter 2: Life And Healing 19
   Plants Respond Directly To 'Ki' 21
   The Reason Why An Indian Man Was Healed Instantly ... 22
   If You Blame A Part Of Your Body, Then You Will Be Punished By It 23
   To Breathe Deeply Is To Live Long 26
   Happy Memories Also Have The Power To Heal The Mind And Body 27
   There Is A Mechanism In The Brain That Makes Us Feel Happiness 29
   If You Leave The Mind In The Now, Things Become Easy 30
   Keeping Our Minds In The Present And Living In The Present 32

For The Energy Of The Cosmos To Work On You, You Must First Relax Your Muscles 33

Chapter 3: Life And 'Sōnen' 37
The Power Of The Image 39
To Picture An Image Successfully 41
The Incredible Power Of The Imagination 43
Marriage Hopes Resurrected. 44
'Sōnen' Can Even Control The Weather 46
Feelings Of Fear Can Create A Frightening Situation 49
If You Wish For A Better Future, Then Live Better Now ... 51

Chapter 4: Life And Hope 53
In Order For A Wish To Become Reality, Repetition Is Necessary. 55
Don't Change Your Wish Whilst In The Middle Of Picturing It 56
The Solution To A Problem Can Be Given To You In A Dream 57
If You Do Not Change What You Are Thinking Deep Down, You Will Not Be Able To Improve Your Health Or Your Finances 58
When We Pray, The Infinite Energy Of The Universe Acts On The Object Of Our Prayers 60
In Order For A Dream To Come True, Try And Imagine You Are Actually Living It 61
For Those Who Are Frightened Of Death, Practise Imagining The Way You Would Ideally Like Your Natural Life To End 63
If You Don't Want To Repeat The Same Mistake Again,

Don't Regret Making The Mistake 65

Chapter 5: Life And Words 67

The Positive And Negative Waveforms Found In Words ... 69

A Technique To Make Sure Your Views Are Taken On Board 71

If What You Think Is Different To What You Do, Your Body Will Become Distorted 73

When We Talk About Our Hopes And Dreams They Become Realized In Words, Making It Hard For Them To Become Reality 75

Start The Day With Positive Words End The Day With A Clear Mind 77

If You Deny Something, Your Capacity Will Diminish 79

There Is No Inherent Good And Evil In Things Themselves. It Is People Who Decide This 81

Chapter 6: Life And The Self 85

On Freedom 87

The Importance Of Deciding Things Yourself 89

Being Critical Of Yourself Can Bring About Unexpected Repercussions 91

Essentially, Human Beings Have No Fixed Self 92

If You Try Something, No Matter How Small, A Path Will Open Up Before You 93

Look With Your Own Eyes! Think With Your Own Head! Live Your Own Life! 96

We Should Not Put So Much Importance On Form 97

Freeing Yourself From Rules and Preferences Will Make It Easier To Live 98

All Answers Can Be Found Inside Yourself.........................99
Not Having Money Can Be Tough, But On The Other Hand, Having Too Much Can Bring Suffering 102

Chapter 7: Life And Living 105
About 'En' (The Bond Between People) 107
If You Don't Want To Feel Failure, Don't Expect............109
Forgiveness 111
Point Out The Bad Points In Children, But Don't Criticize Them 113
Obstacles And Hardships Are Here To Polish The Soul...115
When You Sympathise With Someone, Don't Let Their Grief Take You Over 118
How To Make A Friendship Last Long 120
When Frightened In The Midst Of Darkness, People Seek The Maternal Spirit..122

Chapter 8: Life And Yoga 125
What Is Yoga? 127
Yoga Breathing...128
Yoga Poses..131
The Key And Goal Of Asanas 132
If You Continue Practising Yoga Throughout Your Life, You Will Develop Great Power 133
Practice Yoga With Confidence.......................................135
Yoga And Food 136

Chapter 9: Life And Meditation...141
Why Should We Do Meditation?....................................143

    The Object Of Concentration Should Be Something You Are Fond Of 145

    Yoga Trains The 'Plant' Nerve (The Mind and The Soul) . 151

Chapter 10: The Power Of Life. Methods Of Practice. 159

    A Method To Prevent Oneself From Slipping Into Despair 161

    The Method Of Meditation From The Desert 163

    The Method For Sharpening Your Powers Of Intuition ... 164

    A Method For Boosting Your Level Of Ki 165

    A Breathing Exercise For People Who Find It Hard To Sleep At Night 166

    A Method For Receiving The Energy Of The Sun Into The Body When You Get Up In The Morning 169

    A Pose You Can Do For A Good Night's Sleep 170

    The Way To Use Ki When You Want To Make Your Point Known To Someone 171

    An Easy Way To Relax While Lying Down 172

    An Exceptionally Easy Way To Get Rid Of The Ailments Of The Body 173

Afterword: I Live By Joining The Flow Of The Universe 175

    I Live By Joining The Flow Of The Universe 181

The Translator

Three Years ago, when I was twenty two, I damaged my spinal cord in an accident and became confined to a wheelchair. After leaving hospital, I was very fortunate to be introduced to Mr. Mochizuki and receive therapy from him. When I went to his practice I immediately sensed a calming, healing presence, which I understood as being 'Ki'. I thus realized that Mr. Mochizuki was no ordinary person, but someone who was able to harness this special energy continually and freely. His therapy sessions have continued to help alleviate various painful areas and strengthen my body. Through this direct connection with 'Ki', I am convinced of its existence and recognize the importance of cultivating it through Yoga.

I am very grateful for the trust Mr. Mochizuki has placed in me to write a translation of his book. By translating his words, I have been able to study them carefully and as a result, they have become a constant source of reference and encouragement. In Japanese, Mr. Mochizuki's writing is refreshing and soothing like the effect of 'Ki'. I sincerely hope this translation does it justice and that you may benefit from the book in the same way that I have. Lastly, I would like to thank Mr. and Mrs. Takeda with the translation and Glenda Pritchard for both her help in the final preparation of this book and in bringing it to publication in the UK.

Chapter 1: The Journey Of Life

The Meaning Of Being 'Allowed' To Live

Under pressure from our busy lifestyles, I wonder if there are many of us who truly feel that we are being 'allowed' to live.

When we travel we can distance ourselves from our daily lifestyles and break from the routine of life. In doing this, we awaken our hidden sensitivity so that even as we experience or look at the same things, we will find something new each time. In his book, 'The Divine Code Of Life' (Sunmark Publishers), Professor Emeritus Kazuo Murakami of Tsukuba University states that moving to a new environment can activate dormant genes in the body, causing a sudden noticeable change in a person.

When I was in my twenties, I journeyed from Turkey through Iran, Afghanistan and Pakistan to India using the local buses and trains. It still all remains very vivid in my mind. At first, I was continually critical of my environment. In comparison to Japan and Western society, it was unhygienic, chaotic and unpredictable; you didn't know what was going to happen next.

One day, utterly exhausted from my travels, I walked around the North Indian town of Amritsav, having just crossed the border from Pakistan to India. Here I found beggars, emaciated cows, foul smelling alleyways, and a teeming cacophony of cars, bicycles and rickshaws. I drifted feverishly through the crowds, overcome with exhaustion. Just then, I saw a stern looking pilgrim with a turban, sporting an impressive beard who was milling around in the Square, sword in hand. In front of him, people were washing their hands in a fountain before entering a large building. I learnt from a nearby souvenir seller that inside the building I would find The Golden Temple, and that anyone could go in as long as they washed their feet, entered barefoot, and wore something on their head. I later found out that this was in fact the Head Temple of the Sikh religion. I covered my head, washed my face, hands and feet along with the other people, and followed them inside.

The floor was made of marble, its sharp coldness very pleasant against the soles of my feet. Inside four roofless high walls, a square of marble colonnades surrounded a large lake. In the middle of the lake was an island on which stood a golden temple, shining brilliantly under the intense Indian sun. Cushions lay dotted about in the colonnades, and people used them as they pleased: sitting down on them to meditate, or laying down on them to rest. With the pilgrims, I used the cushion as a pillow and lay down in one of the colonnades. The cool marble felt delightful as it chilled my body from the summer heat. With the gentle breeze drifting in from the lake, I felt my mind and body relaxing for the first time since leaving Turkey. As I lay enjoying this breeze, I found to my surprise tears were streaming down my face. I realized that at that moment I was being healed. That instant I understood that my existence was only possible thanks to this breeze, thanks to Mother Nature and thanks to the existence of every living person.

This realization had deeply affected me inside and from that moment on, the negative thoughts I had of my environment completely vanished.

My Experiences After I Stopped Thinking Negatively

Travelling from Turkey to India, many things annoyed me and made me resentful towards people. As a result, I never got treated well in return. In actual fact, I was treated rather harshly, and not just by human beings. Somehow I felt that dogs, cows and even buses, trains and hotels showed hostility towards me.

Strangely enough, shortly after I stopped feeling resentment towards people, things started to change. This time when I took the train the person in front of me started up a friendly conversation. When the train stopped, he went out and bought me a cup of chai tea from the platform. Another time on the train, a middle-aged man who was sitting in front of me stuck out his tray of lunch and offered me half of it. For some reason or another, people started to behave very kindly towards me.

Again, I experienced another incident when I was buying a boat ticket from Bombay (present day Mumbai) to Goa. After me in the queue was a group of Japanese university students, also buying tickets to Goa. It was around the time when the Beatles were going to India, so it had become a very popular destination for young people and students. After a while, I heard shouting coming from the ticket booth. A man who I guessed was the leader of the group, was protesting about the tickets being too expensive. He began to point in my direction. "That person paid half the amount you're charging us. Why have we got to pay double?" he yelled. "Because that man has the monks' fare", the sari-adorned ticket lady staunchly replied. It was only when I heard this that I realized that she had given me a discounted ticket. At that time I was wearing a long Indian shirt to the knees, with white baggy trousers underneath to keep me cool in the heat. On top of this, with my long hair and beard, and my luggage being just one small pouch, the lady had kindly thought of me as a travelling monk and charged me only half the usual fare. Even though the ladies at the ticket booth weren't particularly efficient in what they were doing, I had not felt a single bit of resentment towards them. As a matter of fact, I had looked upon them favourably.

The experience made me realize that like an underground water system, deep in our minds we are all linked to one source. Therefore, blaming someone becomes the same as blaming oneself. I experienced first hand that when you let go of these negative feelings you start caring for oneself and become tolerant with any situation.

Relying On Intuition

When travelling for a long time, the senses seem to sharpen and the power of intuition gets stronger. When I was in Africa, my intuition helped me a number of times to escape from trouble.

One of these times was in Zaire. I was on a truck, being driven from one village to another. People paid money to get a lift on the back of these trucks, as there were no buses in the area. We finally arrived at the destination at dusk, after being on the road non-stop from five in the morning.

The day before, I had met a Japanese University student and since we were both Japanese, we decided we would feel more secure travelling together. We arranged to leave on the back of one of the trucks early the following morning.

Morning came, and for some reason, I felt hesitant about going. The more I tried to put aside this feeling, the more it grew stronger. Finally, I picked up some courage and decided to follow my intuition. Although I felt bad about letting the student down, I told him to go by himself as something had come up. He therefore left without me.

The following morning, I got on the back of the truck, alone, with a group of African people. The locals were squashed in like sardines, along with the luggage. The road was full of holes and if you didn't hang on tight enough, it felt as though you would be thrown out. It was evening, and as the truck continued its course in the pitch black, a stream of fluorescent objects whistled passed my face. To my amazement, these objects were actually enormous fireflies. Sticking my head out from the back of the truck to have a look around, I saw that we were enveloped in a cloud of these things. It felt as though I was in a dream, drifting in the Milky Way. After some time riding this 'Milky Way railroad[1]', we finally arrived at our destination.

The young guy that had left the day before was waiting for me, but he seemed to be injured. His arms and legs were wrapped in bandages. When I asked him what had happened, he told me that on the previous day his truck had overturned in transit. Many people were injured, including some who had broken their legs, and some who had sustained head injuries. The accident had happened in the middle of their journey, and with great effort, the passengers had to use all their strength to get the truck back up on the road again. It was a long hard slog to finally make it all the way to their destination. I got goose pimples hearing this. I wondered what would have happened if I had ignored my intuition and got on that truck the previous day.

---

[1] 'The Milky Way Railroad' is a well-known novel by the Japanese author, Kenji Miyazawa.

Following one's intuition is I think quite a difficult thing to do. I knew a person who was invited to go shopping by a friend and, even though he somehow didn't feel like going, he reluctantly went. He subsequently got injured in a traffic accident. These sorts of cases where afterwards you think, 'silly me, if only I'd followed my intuition!' are more common than you might think.

One day, during one of my yoga classes, I talked about my experience in Africa and how I had followed my intuition. One of my students who had been listening to my story at the class had just got on the train to go home, but somehow felt uneasy about where he was standing. Thinking that this was his intuition talking, he quickly moved place. Suddenly, before the train had even begun moving, the windows around where he had just been standing shattered, and the passengers around that place were injured from the shards of broken glass.

Getting Rid Of An Attachment To Things

I was in my twenties. From Istanbul I planned to travel to India by land through Iran, Afghanistan, and Pakistan. I stayed in Istanbul for some time before commencing the trip.

I had up to then been collecting interesting coins from my travels. My purse was crammed full of them, and had begun to take the shape of a tennis ball. I was worried about leaving the purse in my shared lodgings, so I took it with me wherever I went. I had planned to travel all the way to India, and the coins had become a bit of a burden. I heard that there was a young couple in the hotel who were Primary School teachers and were collecting coins themselves. I went to them and gave them the whole purse. They were both overjoyed and thanked me profusely, but in fact it was me who wanted to thank them. I remember clearly even now the great sense of relief as I gave the purse full of coins away - it was a real weight off my mind and body.

A Stirring Image In An Ancient Hindi Temple

As I was suffering from acute hepatitis at this time, I had to take rest in the town of Mahabalipuram (modern day Mamallapuram) a suburb of Madras (present day Chennai). There, in a small village facing the sea, was a Hindu temple right next to where the waves were breaking. I was staying in a small hotel in the village. I say hotel, but it was more like a one-story house with five different sized rooms. My room was the space of about six 'jō'[2] and there was a large fan on the ceiling, with long wing-like blades. The room was en-suite and included a young male servant standing by at the door. At the time (twenty five years ago) this cost me five rupees (about 150yen or 75p) for a night.

It got really hot during the day, so I would pass the day lying on my bed with the ceiling fan on and go for walks early in the morning and late in the evening to conserve my energy. After rising in the morning, I would shower, then wash my face, and drink the glass of chai tea brought to me by the servant boy. I would then walk along the sandy path to the beach. The breeze was always refreshing and the sky always a clear blue. On this beach in the Bay of Bengal, there was only one temple dedicated to the Hindu god Shiva. This seaside temple was made of stone, and was enclosed by stone walls. Inside the stone precinct, statues of cows encircled the

---

[2] A 'jō' is the size of a Japanese tatami (a six feet by three feet mat) and is used in Japan to measure the size of floor space.

temple. The cows' faces were indistinct, worn down by the wind. The temple had the same kind of roof as a southern Indian type of pyramid, the Shikara, and was constructed out of an Indian red sandstone. It was said to have been built in the Eighth Century. It too had been eroded by the wind, and parts of it had collapsed onto the beach. I would stand barefoot on the moist sand facing the sea, and wait patiently for the morning sun to rise from the deep blue horizon. Soon the sun would begin to show its face and a wall of light would hit me in the eyes. The sea would begin to sparkle, as though it had been coated in silver dust. The light would reach the black granite columns inside the dilapidated temple. These illuminated wide black columns, or *Linga* as they are known in India, symbols of the god Shiva, would stir me deep inside with their mysterious power.

A Wonderful Experience Of Becoming One With Nature

After standing there for a long time, I would begin to walk along the beach. On the sand small pink empty shells, like little girl's fingernails, were scattered about. The village locals were going fishing in the sea, in primitive dugout canoes- literally hollowed out logs. One after another the men went in and out of the rough, black ink-stained Indian sea. I would watch this scene and then retire to my room in the hotel before the sun became very strong.

In the early evening, when the sun wasn't so intense, I would go for another walk. The village would be filled with the smell of incense and smoke, and the sound of Hindu song. Huge rocks were dotted around the place. I would see these rocks in a stonemason's workshop, being skillfully chiseled into animals such as cows, elephants and lions or temple sculptures. Among other things there were also beautiful reliefs which were made to a high standard of artistry. The workshop would occasionally be crowded with pilgrims as it was a sacred Hindu place.

I would usually climb up the rocky mountains to escape the crowds. At the craggy peak I would look around for a good rock to sit on and gaze out to the horizon. Through the wide spread of marsh and fields I would see a range of mountains veiled in haze. Above this hung the big red evening sun. At this point, on one occasion, an Indian man approached me. I assumed he was probably trying to sell me something. Sure enough, he took out a box containing two baby mongooses and asked me if I wanted to buy them. I waved my hand to tell him I didn't want them. The man left. The cries of the little mongooses gradually diminished to silence.

The sun would sink, inch by inch. The ripe red tomato-like sun would reach the horizon and distort into a slight oval before gradually disappearing. I would watch the sunset with my entire being. When the sun had set, the sky would be dyed a red crimson and it would begin to get dark and a little chilly. On days when the weather was good, while the sun was setting, a similar looking big red moon could be seen to rise up from above the horizon of the Indian sea. When I first saw this phantom-like moon, I mistakenly thought that the sun had began to rise again. As it rose higher into the middle of the sky, it would turn to a brilliant white. After sunset, I would climb down the mountain (making sure I didn't fall) to a restaurant in the village where I would eat supper before retiring to my hotel room. This had all become part of my daily routine.

Spending a whole month in this way I gradually regained my strength. This period of recuperation is an experience I will never forget. One day while returning down the mountain, I decided to walk towards the marshy area. Here, there were paddy fields with interlacing paths. While walking along these paths, I was struck with a wonderful feeling of intimacy. Everything around me including the horizon, the birds flying in the sky, the grass and flowers growing in the paths, the clouds in the open sky, the wind and the smell of dried grass, all seemed familiar to me. An indescribable sense of nostalgia came flooding into my consciousness. This feeling was so intense that floods of tears came pouring down my face. I discovered afterwards that I had experienced a strong case of what is known as *déjà vu*.[3]

Stung By A Scorpion And Thinking Of Home

This was when I was resting in Mamallapuram, a suburb of Madras. Whilst on my way down a mountain, I was stung by a scorpion. It felt as if or as though someone had stuck a needle into the instep of my right foot. Looking around my feet in the dark, I caught a glimpse of a black insect scuttling off behind a rock. The instep of my foot was in extreme pain and began to swell up. Aghast, I shouted out "I've been stung by a scorpion!" I knew that the sting of a scorpion could be fatal, and in a cold sweat, I shouted for help at the top of my voice in the direction of the village. In a panic, I grabbed a passer by and begged for help. Soon three or four villagers had gathered around me. They stood around in bemusement, not knowing what to do. I became frantic. The Indian villagers around me finally began to understand what I was saying

---

[3] Unlike in the West, the Japanese do not use the term déjà vu colloquially.

when I started using the English word 'scorpion' instead of the Japanese word 'sasori'.

I told them that I wanted to go to hospital, but they replied that the English hospital in Madras was now shut. First disbelief, then despair began to take a hold of me. A few of the Indians began to haul me up in my helpless state to take me somewhere. Feeling I was done for anyway, I allowed these people to do what they thought was best. The villagers led me to the house of their medicine-man. Inside the dimly lit house was a sculpture of a portly looking elephant sitting cross-legged. A middle-aged Indian man was offering a green leaved herbal remedy to the elephant god. After saying a prayer, he put all the leaves in his mouth, chewed on them then spat them out on his hand. He then spread this dark green herbal mixture evenly on my swollen instep and wrapped it with a bit of cloth ripped from a handkerchief. Gesturing with his hands and body, the medicine-man assured me strongly that I was going to be fine. Despite all of this, I still felt extremely anxious.

I returned to my hotel room, nursing my throbbing foot, afraid that I wasn't going to make it to see the next day. To my relief the pain subsided and the swelling went down after three days. I strongly felt then that if I was to die, I would wish it to be at home in Japan.

In later years, I visited France travelling from Paris by tour bus to the Loire valley. The guide at the time was a middle-aged French man, but he could speak fluent Japanese in the *Kansai* dialect. He had been brought up in the Japanese town of Kobe, and attended a Japanese primary school before moving back to France before the Pacific War. "Even salmon return to the river of their birth to lay eggs and then to die" he said. "Being elderly and suffering from illness, I similarly wished strongly to return to my birthplace of Kobe. I went back a few years ago but the only thing that was the same as before was the pond behind the church" he said, laughing. As he said this I could sympathise with him since I suddenly recalled when I was stung by the scorpion in India how strongly I felt; that if I was to die, I would wish to be in my birth-place in Japan.

It was only because of being ill on my trip that I was able to experience this. I view it as a gift from my illness and for that I am grateful.

In The Desert, Knowledge Becomes Wisdom

From my time in the desert, I learned that experience transforms knowledge into wisdom. It is important to be knowledgeable, but simply to have one's head crammed full of facts is no use at all. Wisdom comes when knowledge becomes useful. For example, even if someone knows all there is to know about driving a car, if he doesn't have any actual experience of driving, then he won't be able to drive.

If someone therefore has no experience of doing something, then the knowledge he has of it will remain nothing more than simply knowledge. However, this knowledge will bear the fruit of wisdom through experience. This wisdom will then work with the knowledge, using it in everyday life. Therefore, despite our fear of making mistakes, we must not avoid experiencing things. The experience of making a mistake becomes a valid lesson which remains engraved in the mind.

The wisdom which can be applied to people's everyday lives is the most useful. This wisdom could also be seen as a vital 'life power'. While travelling in the desert I was always struck with admiration when I encountered it. For example, the people who live in the desert use a leather pouch water bottle called a 'gelba'. The gelba is a bag made from the carcass of a sheep with its head and four limbs cut off, and the skin turned inside out. Water is then put into this 'buckskin' bag and the holes from the neck and four limbs are tied up with string. The water from my polyethylene water bottle was warm and didn't taste good. However, the water the desert people were carrying and drinking from the gelba bag was surprisingly different from what I expected. Even when untying the cord from the sheep's neck in the searing midday heat, the water that came out was delicious and chilled as if it had just come out of the refrigerator.

Initially, I was very mystified as to why this water was so cold, but after a while I worked out the reason why. The water inside seeps out of the pores of the buckskin and evaporates. In this way the water in the wet black leather bag loses heat and stays cold. To be able to drink cool water in the searing heat of the desert was, I thought, an ingenious bit of applied wisdom.

Once, I was given a very thin slice of watermelon. Although at first I thought how stingy the guy was to give me such a thin slice, when I placed it in my mouth I was very surprised to find it deliciously cold. Here was another great example of applied wisdom. Through evaporation, the dryness of the desert took heat from the thinly sliced watermelon, making it cold.

Another time, I went looking for water with some indigenous people in the desert. In this vast expanse of dried land, it didn't seem there could be any water about. After some time, we came across a big crevasse in the ground. Holding on to the jutting out rocks we climbed down this fifty-metre precipice to the bottom. Here, at the base of this rocky cliff, water was filtering through, dripping down in regular time into a pond. I saw traces of sheep dung which told me that shepherds must be bringing their sheep here to drink the water. In order to survive the desert, people had discovered water in the crevasse by applying wisdom gained from experience over a long period of time.

Life Revolves Like A Wheel

Right now, I am eating lunch in a restaurant in the countryside in Southern India. In this restaurant, the wooden tables shine from spilt curry soup. The customers - all Indian men fill all four tables. When I order, a roughly cut banana leaf is put on the table in front of me, and a portion of curry, rice and a few vegetables is placed on top. I see the other customers all skillfully mix and scoop up the food into their mouths using their fingertips. Once a meal is finished and the banana skin's purpose has been utilized, the restaurant owner picks it up and flings it outside into the road. Without any hesitation, the cows in the street come to eat it, picking it up with their long tongues and tucking into their mouths before sauntering off again. There are always two or three children pursuing the cow, waiting for the dung, which is tussled over and picked up with their bare hands. The cow-pat is then shaped into a flat circle and dried out until hard for use as fuel for cooking.

In the countryside in India, people don't normally use the toilet. It seemed that, outside the house, it didn't matter where people did their business. Even so, in this village, I didn't see any human excrement lying around. I soon found out why. When I was about to add my contribution to the street, a parent black pig almost identical to a wild boar came with ten little piglets in tow to eat it. Since if I was to do it here I would probably have my rear licked by these animals, I hesitated and while doing so, an Indian man approached, and pointed to a better place. At this place I'm told to go, I see that there are raised stones for the feet. Perched on these there would be no fear of being licked by the pigs. In this way, all human excrement is cleared up by these black wild boar-like pigs and piglets.

Under the scorching sun, a cow came slowly towards me, pulling a cart along the road. As I watched the cow from my seat in the restaurant, I recalled a similar scene in the Japanese countryside where I was growing up as a child. The upward pointing horns of the cow, the loose skin hanging underneath the horns, the bony bumps on the shoulders. Each rib could be seen clearly on the trunk of this big, gnarled grey cow. The cart led by this cow was filled with a mountain of dry hay and the big wooden wheels made a constant creeking sound as they slowly rolled on the parched ground.

In India, the cow has been treated as a sacred animal since ancient times. The belief that the cow is a god is said to have originated before the Arians invaded, with the Indus civilization. The cow-drawn carts we see today have hardly changed from those from as much as four thousand five hundred years ago excavated in the Harappa and Monjodaro remains. No doubt it is because the cow is an extremely important animal - a vital source of food and transport that it has been revered, since ages past, as a sacred animal by the Indian people. With this in mind, I looked at the cow and cart passing by. Four thousand five hundred years this emaciated cow has been pulling along this cart, with the big wooden wheels moving slowly along.

While staring vacantly at this scene I felt it enter and revolve around in my mind. The banana skin, its role as a plate fulfilled, gets eaten by a cow then turns into cow dung, then fuel, then ash, then fertilizer for a plant, giving fruit to a banana again. In this way it follows a cycle. I can also imagine the cyclic existence of a star. After the peak of its lifetime, a star diminishes in power, eventually expanding at the end of its life and exploding. Turning into dust, it reforms, giving birth once more into a new star.

I wondered if in fact the Ancients were trying to convey this message through the wheels of the cart dragged by this cow. I got the strong realization that the expression 'reincarnation' was born from the wheels of the cow-drawn cart. This is why the wheel of life representing the six states of existence reappears frequently in the statues of the Hindu temples, the gates of the Tibetan temples, in the Tanka (Indian scrolls) and other places.

I thought of these things in my travels, and with realization, felt an enrichment of Self.

Chapter 2: Life And Healing

Plants Respond Directly To 'Ki'

I first discovered the effect Ki has on plants when the ones in my room where I had started to practise Ki therapy and Yoga became noticeably invigorated and full of life. However, it was in a hospital room where I experienced a plant's direct response to Ki.

A man who came to see me occasionally for Ki therapy asked if I could treat his father who was ill in hospital. I was a little hesitant because I had heard that his father, an ex-bank clerk, was very stuck in his ways and would definitely not be accommodating for something as unexplainable and new as Ki. Finally, giving in to his son's insistence, I went to visit him at the hospital.

When I entered the room, a very difficult looking bank clerk was lying on his bed. He looked at me in disdain. "I'm now going to put Ki into your back so please lie a bit to your side" I told him. In the presence of his son he reluctantly obeyed, muttering "I don't believe in Ki you know". Twenty minutes into the therapy the man suddenly started to shout. "The flowers! The flowers are..!" I looked round at the vases of flowers on the window ledge and by the wall. There were many of them, brought, I assumed, by well-wishers. The flowers and leaves of the tulips and hyacinths were full of life and were standing tall and erect. I was astonished. When I entered the room I was sure the flowers on the windowsill were withered with broken stems from being there for many days. "That is incredible", muttered the ill father, staring at the flowers which looked as if they had all straightened their necks. Once he had seen these plants, the sick man meekly let me continue treating him.

His son told me that from then on, everyone who visited him was given a very detailed account of what had happened to the plants. And soon after, I was invited by the father himself to treat him again.

The Reason Why An Indian Man Was Healed Instantly

I am extremely moved when I am able to witness the mysterious power of human healing. Here is one of those occasions.

One day, an Indian man came to my practice. He was a stout looking gentleman in his fifties with a tightly bound turban round his head and a fully-grown beard. I assumed from the Turban that he was a Sikh. Whilst fixing a window frame on the second floor of his house, he had lost his balance and fallen down with the ladder. From the fall, he received a heavy shock to his left shoulder joint which had hit hard on the ground, and was now too painful to move. He had gone to hospital and had an X-ray, but it showed nothing out of the ordinary. Massages, physiotherapy, osteopathy, chiropractics and acupuncture followed, but to no avail, and for the past six months, he had not been able to move his left arm. He had come to my practice after being recommended by a Portuguese relative whose back pain had disappeared in one sitting. His English friend from work came along as well since he was interested to see how the therapy was done.

First I got the Indian man to sit down on a chair and had a look at his neck and shoulder. When I touched his neck, he asked "Should I take my turban off?" "There's no need" I replied, thinking that this would be a bit troublesome for him. "Stand up please" I said, as I also wanted to take a look at his spine. As I asked him to do this, an amazing thing happened: The Indian man lifted his left arm up high with no effort without even realizing he was doing it. The Englishman pointed at him with an excited "Wow!" The Indian man then looked at his up-raised arm with a rather confused expression on his face. "It's ninety nine percent back to normal", he said. I was also very surprised. Most likely, because of my poor English pronunciation, the Sikh had mistaken my command of "*stand* up please" for "*hand* up please!" He moved his arm this way and that. "Your therapy is amazing" he said, deeply impressed.

Since he had such a big fall, the belief that it would thus be very hard for him to be cured must have entered into his subconscious mind. I find that it is often the case that when an idea enters the subconscious it takes firm root there and no matter what therapy one does the symptom subsequently becomes very difficult to get rid of. I believe that my misheard words had slipped into a blank space in the Indian man's mind, and without thinking he had raised his left arm up.

This case of the Sikh taught me that to be cured from any illness you must be liberated from the negative thoughts that are rooted in your subconscious.

If You Blame A Part Of Your Body, Then You Will Be Punished By It

I think all of us have parts of our bodies that we like and parts that we dislike. If we blame and deny the parts that we dislike, we will receive punishment from these parts in return.

Once, an Italian classical ballet dancer came to my place, saying she had sprained her right ankle. My therapy made it a lot better, and she went home happy. However, after a few weeks, she returned again, saying that this time in practice she had hurt her knee. A week later she came back yet again, saying that this time she had lost her balance and hit her hip.

This dancer didn't just dislike her own right foot - she hated it. She liked her left foot, but when it came to her right foot she even said of it that she wanted to "cut it off and throw it away." A few days before any Ballet company auditions, she would always trip up on her right foot and injure herself unexpectedly and as a result ruin the opportunity. I could therefore sympathize with her feelings to a certain respect. I made a suggestion. "Your right foot is part of your body, right?" "If you didn't have your right foot, your life would change dramatically. Seeing it is such an important part of your body, how about if you started showing it more consideration and gratitude?"

As I said this, I suddenly remembered a young man who had come to see me earlier. He had come to my practice saying that he had problems with his stomach. As I listened to this young man's story, I began to realize that out of all his body, he hated his stomach the most. Since it had always caused him trouble, he had began to criticize it and call it names. I guessed that the root of the stomach problems lay in the way he conducted his mind. He was always dissatisfied and critical of the food he ate, and it was becoming a habit. As a result, even though the food was going down, his stomach wasn't able to work properly and felt uncomfortable. Consequently, he was constantly complaining about it. This problem is not unique to this young man but is in fact apparent in many people who have stomach problems. They are often dissatisfied with the food they eat at home and complain about it, saying "not this again" or "ugh, this tastes horrible" when they eat. Normally when the food enters the body, both the stomach and the intestines work extremely diligently, the stomach to digest the food and the intestines to absorb the goodness. However, if one has a complaint or is dissatisfied with something, the stomach and intestines will not work well. There is an Islamic saying "Eat when you are angry and good food will turn into poison." On the other hand, if you are grateful for what you eat, your stomach will react accordingly and function well.

I advised the young man to stop admonishing his stomach and to start feeling gratitude towards it when eating. If he started doing this I told him, he will get better. Sure enough, the young man's stomach problems improved a great deal just from following my advice and changing his way of thinking.

When the Italian woman heard this story about the young man, she stopped feeling resentful towards her right foot and instead started to treat it better. I then told the woman to relax each morning and night, and to imagine being able to move her body easily and comfortably. She did so, and ceased to receive problems from her right foot. The same reasoning can be applied to people and companies or organizations.

Those who deep down criticize or feel resentment to their company (or organization) will unexpectedly be punished in return. This could be in the shape of a cut in salary or a demotion. It can also take the shape of being given uninteresting jobs or being transferred around the company. In a worse case scenario, it could mean getting fired. For those who are hoping this won't happen to them must first get rid of any negative feelings they have about their company. They must then decide in the quiet of their heart what they would like their role in their company to be. They should then imagine this as reality every morning and night.

It is important to paint an image of how one would like to be in one's company not just once or twice a day, but continually through the day. When you do this everyday, the waveforms emitted from this created image will be worked on by the universe. After this, all that is left to do is to receive the end result.

To Breathe Deeply Is To Live Long

We are pretty much unaware of our breathing when we go about our daily lives. From the first cry at birth, we breathe naturally without thinking. However, this natural breathing later becomes fast, short, shallow, rough and unsatisfactory because we are unable to relax. When we look at a beautiful view, our breathing naturally becomes steady and relaxed. When we are deep in concentration, our breathing becomes slow and long. Contrary to this, if we are walking along the street at night and a friend creeps from behind and startles us with a shout, our breath naturally quickens and gets rough as if we are breathing from our shoulders. This also happens when we feel emotions such as lust or anger.

We can see from this that there exists a regulated relationship between our breathing rate and the state of the mind. We can calm and relax the mind by controlling the breathing and taking long, slow breaths. Furthermore, by breathing deeply, we will live longer.

This reminds me of a book I've read, 'Autobiography of a Yogi' by Paramahansa Yogananda (Self-Realization Fellowship

Publishers). In it, it tells us that a human being breathes on average eighteen times per minute, whereas the restless monkey breathes thirty two times. Creatures with long life spans such as the turtle or the snake breathe much less than humans. The big turtle, said to live for about three hundred years, breathes as little as four times a minute. It seems that in the natural world, the longer the period of respiration per minute, the longer the life span.

As humans, we should first breathe out slowly from the stomach. Exhaling should always come first. In Japanese, the word for 'breathing' is 'kokyū'. The 'ko' part of the word means to 'exhale' and the 'kyū' part means 'to inhale'. It is interesting to note that the order for the two parts is 'ko' then 'kyū', not 'kyū' then 'ko'. When one is exhaling, it is important to concentrate on the breath so that it becomes long and slow.

I have also discovered from recent medical research that when one exhales, the sub sympathetic nerve is stimulated. This is why those who are tense and cannot relax should exhale slowly from the bottom of the stomach, concentrating on their breath. After exhaling, simply let the air naturally enter the lungs, without making a forced effort to inhale. After repeating this many times, the sub sympathetic nerve will start working, and the tension in your body will disappear.

Happy Memories Also Have The Power To Heal The Mind And Body

Whilst I was transmitting Ki into the head of a male patient of mine, he informed me that he could see an image behind his closed eyelids.

"I can see it as clearly as watching it on a colour TV", he said. "What kind of scene do you see?" I asked. "I'm at primary school. It's spring, after the harvest, and I'm standing on a paddy field which has been ploughed by a pitch fork. My friends and I are divided into two groups and are throwing clods of earth at each other."

It appeared that this period was the happiest in his life. When the session finished, he opened his eyes, and repeated how fun it was while getting up. He then realized that the pain he was previously suffering from had vanished. From this I realised that the happy memories and images that he was visualizing had the power to rebalance his body.

In fact, we are continually experiencing this in our daily lives: when we are in good spirits and think back to something, the memories are usually happy ones. Contrary to this, when we are in low spirits, we tend to think of unhappy memories. When the flow of Ki is good in our bodies and we are in good spirits, it seems that good memories naturally spring up to the surface.

There are also people who burst out laughing when I am applying Ki to them. Clutching at his belly, one person laughed out loud for over an hour, "This is strange. Why am I laughing? It's not like anything's funny!" he said.

I found this amusing and started to laugh with him. "Come to think of it, I haven't laughed for three years. I probably laughed three years worth just now," he said afterwards. After his laughing stint the pain he had been experiencing left him and his condition improved considerably.

There has recently been a lot said on the benefits of laughing. It eliminates pain, strengthens the immune system, and prevents cancer. The list goes on. In fact, an American journalist named Norman Cousins cured himself from Collagen disease through laughter. He has recorded his experiences of fighting his illness in his book, 'Anatomy of an illness as perceived by the patient' (Iwanami Shoten Publishers). Laughing can also eliminate feelings of uneasiness between people.

When laughing, one loses tension in the body. If you look at Sumo wrestlers or boxers before a match, no one seems to be laughing. Similarly, the reason we find a laughing person welcoming is probably because we know instinctively that that person will not attack us.

For those of you who have recently forgotten how to laugh, please look into the mirror and try laughing. Once you have remembered how to laugh, then your human relationships will undoubtedly improve, and your physical state will also get better.

There Is A Mechanism In The Brain That Makes Us Feel Happiness

Thanks to the recent research of Dr. Susumu Tonegawa, the Nobel prize winner in Physiology or Medicine, it has been demonstrated that there is a mechanism in the brain that feels happiness. According to Professor Tonegawa, when someone concentrates hard to fulfill a task or role, irrespective of its size or how much money is involved, his brain experiences happiness. Furthermore, once a goal has been met, usually another goal follows, initiating further experiences of happiness. If this is the case, we can ascertain that those who have no goals in their lives do not experience happiness.

Dr Shigeaki Hinohara, a ninety-two year old Chairman and practicing doctor at St Luke's International hospital, says that the one downside about getting old is the lack of things to do when elderly. Those who are unhappy and who have uninteresting lives should set goals, however small, and concentrate fully on them. It is highly likely that if you do, your brain will experience happiness, as the feeling of fulfillment in completing a goal will surpass any drug, no matter how effective.

If You Leave The Mind In The Now, Things Become Easy

I think that everyone has experienced that feeling of being driven to the wall by something; as though they are being hunted down. You can't stop thinking about a particular thing and as a result it makes you feel trapped and chokey.

I experienced this feeling once when my work schedule was chock a block and for over a month I worked from nine in the morning to nine-thirty at night. After two or three days, the thought of another month sitting here day in day out confined to a room crept into my mind and I started to find it hard to breathe. My chest stayed tight even while sleeping.

That evening I had a strange dream. I was doing some sweeping in a large garden with a bamboo rake. I was a young monk in training, and the garden seemed to be inside a temple enclosure. The freshly swept sandy ground showed an ordered pattern, like the scales on a fish. A Sennin (a supernatural hermit) appeared, and asked "How many times have you swept the garden?" "Eighty-eight times", I replied. The Sennin shook his head as if to say "Not yet", and left. The next day after I had swept the temple garden, the Sennin returned again to ask me how many times I had swept it. When I told him, he shook his head again, and left as before. This continued every day until one day I started to concentrate carefully on every action I made, and became totally absorbed in sweeping the ground. My forehead glinted with large beads of sweat. At that point, the Sennin appeared and asked me the same question as before. This time my mind was fixed on each individual sweep. The moment was everything. Instinctively I replied "Once". At that moment, the Sennin, nodding in approval, disappeared and was never to be seen again.

When I awoke from the dream, I stopped thinking about things in the future. This moment is all that counts. By putting the mind into the moment, it becomes everything. There is no difference between one day and one month. When I was able to think like this, my breathing immediately became very relaxed.

Our minds are always swinging from the past to the future, which is why we experience anxiety and suffering. By entrusting our minds to the present, we can concentrate solely on the action in hand, or on our breathing. Every image we see should be engraved in our minds moment by moment. If we do this we can keep our minds in the present. Success in doing this will, I am certain, give release to any feelings of anxiety, and will allow you to relax.

Keeping Our Minds In The Present And Living In The Present

What exactly is the meaning of 'living in the present?' To live in the present, you must keep your mind only in the now; in this present moment.

So are there those who do not have their minds in the present? There are, in fact, quite a few. I realized that most of the people who were suffering from some ailment or another and came for treatment to my practice, had their thoughts dwelling not on the present, but on some unpleasant experience in the past.

There are also those who try and escape their unfortunate situation by thinking constantly about the good times in the past and so lose their mind's vitality in the present. Additionally, there are those who, because of worrying too much about the future, have their minds lodged there instead of in the present.

In Japanese Tea Ceremony, a method is taught to control the mind. In order to taste the tea properly, one must have their mind in the present. If one is worrying about the future or keeps thinking about the past, then one cannot properly discern the taste or aroma of the tea.

When the mind rests in the present, one can feel the warmth of the tea bowl, smell the aroma, and experience the bittersweet aftertaste. If one's mind is not in the present however, there is no appreciation like this of the tea: the tea is merely drunk. Once the tea bowl is put down, even if one wishes to taste the tea again, there will be none left in the bowl to drink. This is 'Ichi gō ichi e' (literally 'One meeting in a hundred years', meaning one should cherish the moment). We can apply this to Life itself. Even though the important time called the Present is given to us, if our minds are not in the here and now, then we cannot taste or enjoy living. Life becomes merely the passing of days and months. When approaching Death, simply regretting that one didn't really live life will not turn back the hands of time.

To avoid such regretful thoughts, it is important to put the mind in the Now and live in the Present. If one concentrates on one's breathing, one's mind will immediately return to the Present. Feel the slow exhalation and the inhalation with an empty mind. This is all one needs to do. Then, keeping the mind fixed in the Present, one can do the thing one most wants to do at that time.

That is how to keep one's mind in the Now and thus live in the Present.

For The Energy Of The Cosmos To Work On You, You Must First Relax Your Muscles

In the Universe, there exists a limitless power – the power that created it in the beginning of Time. For this limitless power to work on us, it is necessary for us to relax our muscles. By relaxing our muscles, we can become relaxed in both mind and body, and by doing so become one with the Universe. We know through experience that when we get nervous our muscles tighten, and that when we release the tension in our muscles, we can relax.

So what really is this relaxation? The English word 'relax' comes from the words 're' and 'lax'. 'Re' means in Latin 'again' and 'lax', 'to loosen up'. 'Relax' therefore means in

Latin 'to loosen up again'. So what is it exactly that we 'loosen up again'?

Before we get to that, let us look at the word with the opposite meaning, 'tension'. According to Transpersonal Psychology, from the moment we learn how to speak and see the world, we start to feel tense. The English word 'tense' comes from the Latin word meaning 'time'. Since the other meaning of tense is 'to tighten up', it follows that if the concept of time disappears, inevitably tension also disappears. Furthermore, it implies that only when a state of mind is achieved where time does not exist, can real relaxation be felt. This state of mind where time is irrelevant is the same as the state of mind of babies before they learn to speak. It is equivalent to the world of animism.

If we follow this line of thought, then the 're' from the word 'relax' means to go back once again to the original consciousness where there is no time, in other words to the Universe. To relax is therefore to become one with the Universe.

So what does one need to do to release tension in the muscles? There is a technique that can be learnt which I will now show you.

This method can be practiced anywhere at any time, so please follow it when you can. When you have memorised the method, please start by doing it lying down, then later on you can begin doing it sitting up.

1- Wear comfortable, loose clothes and lie on your back, facing upwards. Gently close your eyes, put your hands in prayer position and point them upwards.

2- First, say to yourself deep down the following: "I am now concentrating on my right leg." Then say to yourself "the toes of my right foot are relaxed", and so on and so forth, in rising order, with the ankle, the calf, the knee, and the thigh. Then say in your mind, "All tension has disappeared from my right leg. It is now completely relaxed." That is your right leg done.

3- Now repeat the process with your left leg.

4- Next say to yourself deep down "I am concentrating on my stomach." Now say "the bowels are relaxed." Repeat this in rising order to the stomach, the heart, the lungs and the neck.

5- Next, say to yourself deep down, "I am concentrating on my right arm." Then say to yourself, "my right-hand finger tips are relaxed", and in rising order do the same to the wrist, the elbow, the shoulder. Now say to yourself, "all tension has disappeared from the right arm. It is now all completely relaxed."

6- Now, in the same way as in (5), release the tension from your left arm.

7- Finally, say to yourself deep down, "I am concentrating on my face." Then say to yourself, "my jaw is loosened, and my teeth are aligned comfortably. The mouth is now relaxed." In rising order do the same to the nose, ears, eyes, forehead and head.

8- Next, say to yourself deep down, "both arms feel heavy and are comfortably attached to the ground."

9- Next, say to yourself, "my back is very comfortably attached to the ground."

10- Next, "both legs feel heavy and are attached to the ground."

11- Next, "The whole body is very comfortably attached to the ground."

12- End by saying, "now my body is completely relaxed", and stay in this comfortable position for five to ten minutes.

When you relax your muscles in this way, your entire body becomes relaxed, and you will be able to access the infinite energy of the Universe. So when you are relaxed like this, make an image of what you wish for yourself. When you do this, your thoughts will become one with the thoughts of the Universe. All you need to do now is just leave it all for the Universe to do. Once your thoughts have been given over to the Universe, the infinite energy of the Universe will work on its own to turn your wishes into reality.

Chapter 3: Life And 'Sōnen'[4]

---

[4] 'Sōnen' is a Japanese term meaning 'belief through imagination'.

The Power Of The Image

Although the word image is used without much thought, in it is hidden an enormous mysterious power. The power of the image is beyond our comprehension.

This is demonstrated in a story taken from the book 'The Heart of Healing' (Turner Publishers) written by William Poole.

Two months before the 1984 Summer Olympics in Los Angeles, the Romanian weightlifter Dragomir Cioroslan suffered a terrible injury during a competition in which he fell on his back, and dropped the 207kg barbell directly onto his neck. Effectively it looked like his glittering sports career had come to an abrupt end. At the time of the accident he was the world weightlifting champion, but his main ambition had been to take the Olympic gold medal. Now it seemed his dream was well and truly over. In spite of this, while lying in bed, unable to move let alone train, he followed instructions from his sports psychologist who told him to continue his training by imagining it in his head. So for eight hours a day, with his eyes closed, he continued to train by using his imagination.

In doing this he recovered quicker than anyone could have imagined, and after as little as two weeks of training he took part in the Los Angeles Olympics, winning the bronze medal.

While in hospital, he had begun by picturing all the movements, every little detail of the training in his head. Until the final action of lifting the heavy barbells, he remembered each part of the process. By repeating this imagery over and over again, it was cemented in his mind.

Once we realize that this incredible power of the imagination is inside all of us, we can surely learn to harness it for our benefit.

If we can make use of the power of the imagination well, we can overcome many difficulties.

In China, people are known to have cured their illnesses by practising Ki exercises. Of these people, it seems that those whose conditions improve the best are those who can use their imaginations well.

For example, there is an account of a patient who, while practicing a Ki exercise, suddenly relived a moment in his past when he was out walking.

A picture came into his mind of a scene bathed in spring sunlight, with ice slowly melting on the surface of a river.

As he remembered his feeling upon watching the ice melt under the spring sunlight, he immediately felt a sense of relaxation, and consequently made a rapid recovery from his illness. With great effect, he had managed to align the image of the melting ice with the image of the illness in his body calming down and disappearing.

As this example demonstrates, the image releases power the moment it is perceived well.

It seems that it is when an image is brought clearly and realistically to mind and especially when an image joins and melts together with a part in the body that a mysterious power starts to work.

It is therefore no good just to think of something vaguely.

To Picture An Image Successfully

When picturing an image, it is important to imagine it in as much detail and as vividly as possible.

How does one imagine like this? Is there a method we can use?

All one needs to do is to imagine using all five senses; sight, hearing, smell, taste and touch.

Once I was invited to Provence by some French people living in Monaco. They were insistent on taking me to their relative's wine museum in a vineyard there. During the trip from Monaco to Provence, we passed florid fields of pale yellow mimosa flowers in full bloom, and the base of a rocky mountain that resembled a small version of the Grand Canyon.

Here I will recount the clearest memory I have of my time in Provence using all five senses.

The car is speeding along a roadway in between wide vineyards. After some time a church spire comes into view. Around the church I can see small villages. There is no sign of anyone around. It is just midday now, and we go and eat at a local restaurant.

After lunch, we walk under the sycamore tree next to the medieval church and decide to take a nap. The trunk of this giant sycamore tree is very thick. Even four adults lined around the tree with arms outstretched can't reach around it. The bark of the tree is rough and in various places it is peeling off.

It is a hot day, but in the shade under the giant tree it is cool and refreshing. I sit down deep into my chair.

The air is dry and the breeze invigorating. It is pleasant against my skin. The breeze brings with it a sweet smell of cypress and I feel its calming effect. I wonder if this is the smell of Provence wind.

Occasionally there are small gusts of wind making the leaves of the sycamore tree up above rustle together. The sky is such a deep blue, I feel it might swallow me up.

In between the sycamore tree and the church is a medieval fountain. There is a delicate sound of running water. The water runs into an oblong water tank for animals to drink. A wood pigeon stops on the edge of the tank, coo-cooing in between drinking.

The sun is strong and the water from the fountain breaks into water droplets, dancing up and falling down without rest, sparkling in the air.

Occasionally the strong sunrays stream through the leaves and make my eyelids flutter. My right arm is out of the shade of the tree and it feels hot.

I take a sip of rosé wine. The wine is cold and sweet, and the bubbles spread out over the inside of my mouth, passing down my throat and settling around my stomach. I start to feel a bit tipsy. I fall into a deep sleep.

How did you feel from reading this?

I was living my experience in Provence again through the use of all five senses in my imagination.

When imagining something I recommend that you too use all five senses so that you re-live the experience vividly in your mind.

The Incredible Power Of The Imagination

People who have been ill for a long time, and who go about their lives constantly thinking and worrying about their illness possibly do so because they have had to continually deal with their illness.

If you say, "imagine yourself to be healthy and full of life" to such people then they will most probably reply that they are unable to do so. They do not think it is possible to conjure up a healthy picture of themselves.

This is perfectly understandable since they have been suffering from the illness for a long time. While I was talking on various subjects to people in this predicament, a middle-aged man said, "Actually, I remember I was in good shape when going mountain climbing with my friends at high school." Just to picture this forgotten memory was enough for him to declare "I think I can now imagine myself healthy again."

From that point on, instead of thinking about his illness, the man created an image in his mind of himself back when he was healthy. Once he was able to do this, he made a surprising improvement.

I have seen this sort of thing happen often.

If you are worrying about an illness you have, you must change your attitude towards it. Ideally, it is best if you can relive the moments of when you were radiant with happiness.

To overcome your illness, it is vital to make the image of a healthy 'you' indelible in the mind.

When I recommend this course of action to people, there are always some who cannot accept it and retort, "you might say that, but life isn't so simple." There are also those who say "even if I picture a wish and cement it in my mind, it will never come true, nor will any effect come from it."

The thing that strikes me when I hear these sorts of remarks is that the person's real feelings are working contrary to a wish they may have. It is these feelings which create the reality for them.

I know of a person who was living in a rented house, and wished to buy his own place. However, in a corner of his heart he knew that such a wish would never be realized on his existing salary. This lack of faith in his wish was what he truly felt and it is this that defined his reality.

Here is another way of looking at it. Say there was a person who congratulated another on his success, but in actual fact resented him and wished he would fail in something. Since down in the deep recesses of the heart is a world without a subject, this wish of failure becomes directed on the person who thinks it. It is this person therefore who becomes the one who experiences failure.

When picturing a wish in the mind it is very important to do so with the fullness of the heart.

Marriage Hopes Resurrected.

A thirty five year-old woman once came to my practice for treatment. She was suffering from ill health but I also sensed that deep down, she had given up on something.

When she had become fully relaxed and began to feel much better, I asked her whether there was anything troubling her. She replied rather unexpectedly, "I don't know if I'll ever be able to marry."

I asked back, "Is there any reason why you can't marry?" and listened as she then began to recount her story.

When she was in her twenties this woman had been to a well-known fortune-teller to find out whether she was to marry or not. The fortune-teller had told her that if she didn't marry in her twenties, then there would be no chance of marrying in her thirties, and only a small chance of marrying in her forties.

She hadn't married in her twenties, and after experiencing a string of unsuccessful relationships with men in her early thirties, the words of her fortune teller had started to loom over her like a dark cloud. She had fully taken to heart the fortune-teller's words and it was clear to see that she had as good as given up on the idea of marriage.

"Since I am now in my thirties any chance left for getting married now has gone", she declared. "If you keep to this belief then you will not be able to marry, but if you detach yourself from these words there is a chance that you will marry in your thirties", I explained.

I proceeded to give the woman the following advice.

"At night in bed before you sleep, think up one by one your requirements for the sort of man you would like to marry. Then say to yourself, I meet this man and we get married. After this try and picture an image of you and your husband married together. Finally give your thanks. Do this every night".

The woman replied somewhat doubtfully. She did not seem particularly convinced.

"You find it difficult because you think you need to put pressure on yourself in order to get married". I said, "There is no need to put effort into it. Just go to sleep once you have finished picturing an image of your future husband. At night, in one revolution of the universe, everything will be done for you. The wavelength of your thought will work on the universe and your wish will be fulfilled. You need not worry about a thing since no effort is needed on your part.

When you get up the following morning, forget all about it, and just go to work as usual. Don't forget to do this", I told her in conclusion, adding, "remember it's not you that does anything; the infinite power of the universe does it all."

She appeared relieved as I gave her this advice. I saw her spiritless face become at once bright and cheerful.

Whether or not she chose to heed my advice was completely up to her. Seven months later, there was a phone call from the woman. Since her voice was cheerful, I assumed she had some good news.

"Hi, this is Mrs.X. Do you remember me? I am now married. It's amazing, it really does work."

This woman had practiced what I had advised every night before going to bed. After doing this for 4 months, she had met someone who fulfilled all of her requirements. After that it had been just a matter of time before they got married.

'Sōnen' Can Even Control The Weather

In 'sōnen', thoughts and image creation are powers that can create reality.

When a waveform from a thought joins with another waveform of the same type, it has the power to become real and affect your surroundings.

When taking my driving test in London, I was shown a clear demonstration of the power that can be generated from one's 'sōnen'.

My 'sōnen' changed the weather.

In the week before my driving exam, I set aside some time each day to lie down, relax and imagine passing the test in the following way.

To start off, the driving instructor has the mark sheet in his hand and is sitting in the passenger seat. I start the car running. The driving instructor then gives me orders one after the other to turn right, then left. I am relaxed, and follow my orders without any trouble.

The driving test is now over, and I'm sitting in the driving seat waiting for the result. In the passenger seat, the driving instructor is marking the sheet. He finishes, sticks his hand out with a smile on his face and says "you've passed." The instructor then takes out a certificate indicating that I've passed and asks me to sign it, telling me that it is carbon paper so I have to write down hard. I take the ballpoint pen off him and sign my name down firmly. My face is happy and smiling.

In this way, every day before going to bed I made an image in my mind in as much detail as possible of what was going to happen. The more realistic and detailed your image is, the more strongly and deeply it is imprinted on your mind. After a week of image training, the day of the exam finally arrived.

The examination place was full of people. Inside, the receptionist was reading out the names of the applicants one after another. When my name was called out I answered promptly. Failure to answer was attributed to bad hearing and resulted in immediate rejection.

So far so good. It was after this, however, that a problem arose.

I gathered from looking at the person before me, that the driving instructor would start the exam by first walking to a car twenty yards (about eighteen metres) away from the front entrance from where he would ask the applicant to read the number plate.

People who could not answer or made a mistake were taken to the rear garden and were asked to try again. If they still couldn't read the number plate correctly then they were given a fail.

I had been very careless in forgetting to have my eyesight tested for my glasses. I hadn't until that time been for a sight test for about ten years. My nearsightedness had definitely worsened in that time. As I waited my turn, I had a go at reading the number plate the examiner was pointing at from behind the window, but could not make it out at all. I've failed, I thought to myself. But immediately after thinking this I remembered that since I had been making an image of the examination everyday for a week, the image of passing was now fully inputted in my mind. I therefore became confident in the belief that somehow it was going to be all right.

Along came my turn. All of a sudden, the sky turned black and a torrent of rain hit the ground.

To avoid getting soaked by the rain, the examiner, who was forced to stand under the porch of the entrance, pointed to a car parked just two or three metres away, and asked me to read the plate. I broke out in a smile. Whether this was fair or not is debatable, but somehow or other I had managed to get through to the next stage. After this point in the exam, everything progressed smoothly just like I had imagined it to.

At the end, the examiner who had been marking in the passenger seat congratulated me. "You've passed" he said. As he handed me the driving certificate to sign with a ballpoint pen, he asked me to press down hard as there was a carbon copy underneath.

What I had pictured in my mind every day had become reality.

After having this experience I am now firmly in the belief that 'sōnen' can also change the weather.

Feelings Of Fear Can Create A Frightening Situation

On the 17th of January 1995, a huge earthquake rocked the city of Kobe, and as many as six thousand three hundred people lost their lives. It was the biggest disaster in Japan since the 2nd World War. Pictures of the disaster areas on television had a huge impact on many viewers. A Japanese woman who lived in London was one of these people. She saw the scenes on TV and couldn't get them out of her mind. As a result, in her daily life, she became always fearful of something terrible happening.

She arrived at my practice suffering from a whiplash injury, apparently the result of a rear end collision with another car.

She had noticed a car advancing at a fast pace in her rear-view mirror but as there was still sufficient distance between them, she had presumed the car would drop its speed. Suddenly however, the fear she had felt while viewing the aftermath of the earthquake and the fear of the car crashing into her merged together and she panicked. As she braced herself in anticipation, sure enough, true to her worries, the car collided hard into the back of hers. The driver of the incoming car was an English man in his seventies.

In the case of this woman, her fear had created the situation.

This works conversely for a different type of people.

There was a family from Kobe who, because of the father's work, relocated to London in December. Originally, they were supposed to move in February or March, but much to their dissatisfaction this was moved to an earlier date. It so happened that because they moved earlier, they missed the Great Kobe earthquake.

Another man who was working as a Japanese business attaché in London was sent out to Japan and just happened to be in Kobe when the earthquake struck. There are also those who suffered accidents associated with the earthquake even though they were living in the safest areas away from it.

All these instances show us that the fear or worry that people hold in their hearts can turn into reality or cause other bad things to happen.

On the other hand, even if a frightening situation develops, if one always feels peaceful or safe, it will pass without one getting hurt.

If You Wish For A Better Future, Then Live Better Now

The present you is a manifestation of your continued 'sōnen' from the past. To put it simply, the present reality is here as a result of what has been done in the past.

It is no different regarding health.

If a person is diagnosed with having diabetes there is undoubtedly a reason behind it. It has come as a result of living an unbalanced life for a long time. The state of health of a person today is a direct result of his/her past.

In the same way, the actions you take and the thoughts you think all contribute to creating your future. You are able, therefore, to foresee to some extent how your situation will be in the future from the way you conduct yourself and the way you live now.

If you care little for your health and spend your days drinking heavily and overeating, then you can predict that soon you will experience problems with your stomach. Caring about your health and treating your body well results in the ability to maintain a good state of health.

Those who wish for a better future and who understand that the present causes the future and accordingly that the future is a result of present actions will know that they must choose a better way to live now.

Chapter 4: Life And Hope

In Order For A Wish To Become Reality, Repetition Is Necessary.

Constant repetition is needed in order for anything to be realized, no matter what it is.

Constant repetition is the most important factor in Yoga and is called Abhyasa. Training is when you repeat the same thing over and over again in order to master it.

Whether it be for sports or for performing musical instruments, progress is made from repeated practice.

In the same way, in order to make a wish come true, it is essential to picture it over and over again in your mind. The infinite energy of the universe starts to work on something once it is repeated.

It is extremely rare for a wish to come true by imagining it only once. If everything immediately went according to our wishes then there would be no more suffering in the world.

It seems that in the world we live in now, the things we wish for rarely come true. It is thus said that the time we have in this world is the only time when we can train ourselves. The very fact that our desires cannot be achieved immediately may be where the value of this world lies.

Furthermore, in my experience, when you start to doubt your 'sōnen' (belief through imagination), your wishes are in fact on the brink of coming true. Yet most people give up one step before this stage.

Take this story, for example. A woman who was working overseas received a job offer in Tokyo as a university lecturer, but the pay was meagre. She had wanted to live in a comfortable place but was worried that the rent would be too much for her. When I heard this I recommended that she create an image of living in a comfortable and spacious flat every night before going to sleep, and through repetition engrave this image on her mind.

After a month I received a phone call from her.

"Even though I've been picturing it every day nothing has happened. Maybe I'm asking for too much. I doubt it will happen now."

"The fact that you have started doubting it means it will happen soon. Just keep continuing with it, don't give up" I replied.

Two days later I heard from her again. This time her voice sounded bright and cheerful. Apparently, the father of her friend had moved overseas because of work, and asked her if she would like to live in his flat, rent-free as long as she kept it clean. This move overseas was likely to be for an extended length of time, so she was able to live there for a long period. In this way, the woman was able to live in a very comfortable and spacious flat just as she had always wanted.

In general, people who have success are those who keep their dreams alive until they are realized. Therefore, in order for your wishes to be fulfilled, please keep creating the image you wish for in your mind.

Don't Change Your Wish Whilst In The Middle Of Picturing It

Once you have started imagining your wish as reality, you should not change it in any way, unless for a very good reason.

What you have imagined as reality in your mind produces waveforms during your sleep, which are acted upon the Universe.

The Universe moves into action as its infinite energy works to gradually realize your wish.

That is why to change the wish while in the process of realization is a huge waste of energy. It means everything has to start from square one again. All the work done by the universe in turning the wish into reality will thus count for nothing.

Those therefore who change their wishes regularly are not just wasting the energy of the Universe, but also making it difficult for their wishes to be realized.

To avoid the chance that you might change it later, it is therefore necessary to choose your wish carefully before you start imagining it.

The Solution To A Problem Can Be Given To You In A Dream

I will relate a story I heard from a woman who comes to my yoga class in London.

The husband of this lady had misplaced his car keys somewhere in the house. He had looked in all the places where he thought the keys could be, but could not find them.

He was in trouble because he had to use the car the next day.

While looking for the keys, the woman remembered the words I had said at yoga practice, "the answers to everything can be found inside your mind."

Before going to bed, she prayed to herself.

"My husband's car keys have been found. Please let me know where they are."

That night the woman saw a dream. In this dream she saw the clothes pegs in the corridor of her house on which the coats were hung. She saw that her husband's car keys were inside the pocket of one of these coats. She saw that there was a hole in this pocket and that the keys had fallen down into the coat.

When she opened her eyes she immediately arose and searched the coat. Just as it had appeared to her in her dream, she found the keys through a hole in the pocket.

Keep in mind that if you ask yourself deep down for the answer to a problem, it may be revealed to you in a dream.

If You Do Not Change What You Are Thinking Deep Down, You Will Not Be Able To Improve Your Health Or Your Finances

Once, I went for a week to Madrid, Spain to practise Ki therapy on some patients.

What I experienced on one day during my trip made me realise fully that unless people change what they are thinking deep down on a conscious or unconscious level, they will not be able to improve their situation.

That day was when, on request from a Japanese woman, I went to treat her Spanish husband who had been off work due to a bad stomach.

He had tried many different treatments but none of them had had any effect.

"Well then, now it's time to try Ki therapy" I enthused, but he made various excuses and stubbornly resisted any such treatment.

His wife was at a loss as to what to do.

Although it was clear his wife wanted me to treat him, after learning more about him from her, I decided not to go ahead.

"It appears that your husband is content with being ill", I told her.

The wife worked for a big Japanese trading firm in Spain and earned a large salary. Even if her husband didn't work, it would not have made much difference to their lives. By having a bad stomach and so being excused from going to work, the husband could look after the children at home. And in spite of his bad stomach he drank alcohol every day.

It was the possibility that his stomach might get better that had been a constant source of worry for the husband.

If his stomach got better, no longer would he be able to miss work and play with the kids, or continue drinking alcohol from the afternoon onwards in the comfort of his home.

It is because he thought these things would be taken away from him that he was determined not to let me treat him.

This man is not the only one, I am sure of that. There are many others who, be it consciously or unconsciously, choose to be ill because it suits them better. This applies not just for illnesses, but also for money.

Some people with money problems probably subconsciously loathe or feel that they want to do away with money.

Hence, when we really want to overcome an illness or relieve a money situation, it is necessary to change what we are thinking deep down.

When We Pray, The Infinite Energy Of The Universe Acts On The Object Of Our Prayers

Is praying merely something that eases our anxieties and makes us feel better about ourselves? Or does it wield a power that can have an actual effect on something?

Research done at a certain American university hospital shows that praying does indeed have an influence on things.

Carefully performed research was carried out using two groups of people. Prayers were made for only one of the groups. The results showed that the people in the group that wasn't prayed for recovered slower from their illnesses than those in the group that was prayed for.

Results carried out by a certain research group in America on seeds of rye also displayed the same results. No matter how many times the experiment was carried out, the probability of sprouting was much higher for the seeds of rye that were prayed for than for those that did not have people pray for them.

From my experience of practising long distance Ki therapy, I believe that these occurrences happen because the infinite energy of the universe works on the object that is being prayed upon. According to the research team in the book, 'Ikigai No Honshitsu' ('The Kind Of Life Worth Living') (written by Dr.

Fumihiko Iida, published by PHP Institute, Inc.), the effects of praying can be analysed in the following way.

1- The distance between the prayer and the object is of no consequence to how effective the prayer is.

2- The effects are greater for people who pray often than for those who only pray occasionally.

3- Rather than to pray aimlessly for all the people suffering from illness in the world it is much more effective to pray for a specific person or specific people. Having said that,

4- even if the amount of people prayed for increases, the effect is not lessened.

Therefore, even if you are far away from your family or friends and cannot go and meet them directly, do not despair. You can make the Universe work its infinite energy on anyone you wish through prayer.

Remember that when praying, it is important to picture clearly the person we are praying for, and to have conviction in our prayers.

In Order For A Dream To Come True, Try And Imagine You Are Actually Living It

There was an occasion when a young doctor came to my house in London from Japan after hearing about me through a friend of his.

He had just graduated from a medical college, and his dream was to work in a healthcare centre abroad. In order to achieve this goal he had decided that he would need to study at the London School of Hygiene & Tropical Medicine.

He went for an interview with a professor at the University. The professor told him that there would be no problem for him to study there, but pressed him over whether or not he could afford the tuition and accommodation fees. He replied that he could, but there was doubt in his mind. Even if he went on night duty as a doctor every day of the week, it would take years to save up the kind of money needed to pay the fees.

When the young doctor finished speaking, I recommended that he actually lived his dream in his mind every night before going to bed.

"Imagine you are in the experiment room in the London School of Hygiene & Tropical Medicine, holding a beaker and doing research, as if you are really there", I told him.

The young doctor went back to Tokyo and practiced this every day, picturing his wish and imagining everything as if it was actually happening.

During this period, he contacted me occasionally to say that he wasn't saving any money and that he was worn out and doubted things were able to get better. When he said these things, I would urge him to keep the faith and not to give in, to continue keeping the image of his wish in his mind's eye.

Sure enough, one year later, he was awarded a scholarship from a Japanese company based in London and was able to get a place at the tropical disease section of the Faculty of Medicine at the University of London.

Further to this, he was also fortunate enough to live at the Halls of residence in the residential area of Hampstead in London.

This was located close to where my Yoga classes are held, and once a week he was able to attend.

Perhaps due to improved concentration from doing the yoga breathing exercises, his studies went very well. Whereas it would usually take someone several years to complete a Masters degree it took him little over a year.

Immediately after graduating, he applied to go to Cambodia as a PKO dispatch doctor. He got the job, and in doing so, fulfilled his dream.

Several months later, I received a Christmas card from Cambodia. Underneath a picture of the rainy and dry seasons of Cambodia was a note from the young doctor, telling me how he was continuing to practice yoga breathing exercises everyday so as not to get ill.

For Those Who Are Frightened Of Death, Practise Imagining The Way You Would Ideally Like Your Natural Life To End

If you persevere with your 'sōnen', the things you wish for will come true.

The mind houses the infinite energy of the Universe and so holds the power to make thoughts reality.

We often worry about the future, wondering what would happen if we became senile or bed ridden or if we slipped into a vegetative state and so on and so forth.

Worrying about these things on a day-to-day basis will not prevent them from happening. In actual fact, worrying about them may conversely make them come true.

I always imagine my own natural death in the following way.

I reach old age after a long and healthy life. I am still alert in mind and can manage things on my own without anyone's help. In fact, I am also able to help others a little with their things.

Two days before the end of my life, the physical signs that tell me I am about to die appear, and realising that the time has come to go into the other world, I tidy myself up, spread my futon out on the floor and lie down to go to bed. In my mind I think, "death in this world means birth in the other world, death in the other world means birth in this world," and with this thought in mind I start to become relaxed. When one relaxes, a high level of beta-endorphins are secreted in the brain. As this happens, any fear I have in my mind vanishes, and a sense of exhilaration comes over me. In this feeling of rapture I step into the other world. Someone comes to my pillow side but by then I have already peacefully passed away.

I practise imagining something along these lines. For those who worry about death, imagine the ideal way you would like to pass away, (using my description as a reference if need be), and practise this continually.

No doubt your 'sōnen' will be worked on by the infinite energy of the Universe and your ideal way of dying will become a reality.

If You Don't Want To Repeat The Same Mistake Again, Don't Regret Making The Mistake

Generally in this world, it is encouraged to feel remorse over making a mistake to prevent the same mistake being made again.

However, it is debatable whether or not this is necessary for us in everyday life.

Under 'regret' in the dictionary, it says 'to consider past actions and look at them in a critical light'. In other words, feeling regret means we are turning the mistake over and over again in our minds. This leads us to repeat the same mistake again.

A housewife once told me a story about her son.

One year her son took part as a member of the relay team on sports day, but during the race dropped the baton on the pass over. As a result his team came last. He put all the blame on himself for losing the race and deeply regretted dropping the baton. Once again the following year he took part in the relay on sports day but proceeded to drop the baton again, the second time in a row.

After making the mistake the first time, instead of dwelling in regret over dropping the baton, he should have imagined himself taking the baton cleanly and running into the lead.

Another story concerns a certain female pianist. She deeply regretted making a mistake at a concert but made the same mistake again at her next performance even though she had made a special effort not to.

Instead of feeling regret, this pianist should have imagined herself performing without any mistakes.

My thoughts from these stories are as follows. If you experience failure, look at it as just a one-off occurrence. Instead of feeling regret or remorse over your actions, imagine yourself doing a successful job of whatever it is that you are doing, and you will not make the same mistake again.

Chapter 5: Life And Words

The Positive And Negative Waveforms Found In Words

Matter can be broken down indefinitely to atoms and molecules, and further still down to nuclei, electrons and elementary particles.

Recently, even smaller particles called quarks are said to exist. These quantum particles are said to be closer to energy than matter and behave like waveforms. If the energy joining these minute particles is strong they form together to create a hard substance. If the energy is weak then a soft substance is formed. We can say therefore that ultimately everything in the universe is formed from the oscillating waves from quantum particles.

In the same way words too have their own waveforms.

The word 'thanks' for example, has a positive waveform while the word 'idiot' has a negative waveform.

There is a collection of photos of crystallized water called 'Messages From Water' by Dr. Masaru Emoto (Hadō Kyōiku Sha Publishers) which shows this.

In this book there is a section which I found particularly interesting. It shows photos of a glass container which had been labelled by a word processor with certain words and left overnight in a freezer. Water had been poured into the glass container the night before and had turned into ice. The ice in the container with positive words on the label such as 'thank you', 'love', 'gratitude', 'soul', 'angel' 'shiyōne' (Japanese for 'let's do it') and 'beautiful' had formed exquisitely and symmetrically like a snowflake.

However, the ice that had formed in the container with negative words like 'idiot', 'disgusting', 'kill', 'devil', 'Satan' and 'shinasai' ('I demand you to do it') was ugly and distorted.

To see in this collection of photos such clear evidence to suggest that everyday words, which we use without much thought, have their own individual waveforms was very surprising to me.

On one occasion, a housewife came and asked me for some advice. Her plea went something along these lines.

"In the evening when my husband comes home from work, the first thing he says is 'I'm tired'. Even though I was feeling happy and energetic up to that point, when I hear these words I immediately start to feel tired myself. The same happens to my daughter also. What can I do to stop this happening?"

After explaining to the housewife how words emit different waveforms, I told her,

"In the words 'I'm tired' there are negative waveforms that induce or increase tiredness. This is the reason why when you hear these words you are affected by them and become tired."

I then told her to try asking her husband to change what he says when he comes back home to something positive.

Fortunately, her husband at once responded to his wife's plea and thus no more did she have to endure the negative waveforms emitted from the words "I'm tired."

A Technique To Make Sure Your Views Are Taken On Board

In everything on earth there is polarity.

If you measure the voltage of an eggshell by making a hole in the top and bottom of the egg and connecting a voltmeter to it, the top will measure positive and the bottom negative. In the same way, you can measure positive and negative on a sweetcorn kernel. The earth itself also has a north and a south pole.

Human bodies too have polarity. The right-hand side of the body is positive and the left-hand side is negative. Also, the top half of the body is positive, and the bottom half, negative.

For the arms, energy goes out of the right arm and comes in from the left arm.

For the eyes, energy goes out of the right eye and comes in from the left eye.

Once we know that polarity exists like this in the human body, we can use it accordingly.

For example, when you really want to be understood you should make your plea while staring intently with your right eye at the left eye or left side of the body of the person you are talking to. If you do so, the person, regardless of his point of view, will probably start to agree with you.

The following story illustrates this well.

A young man in his thirties who worked in London on transfer from his main office in Japan once told me,

"Whenever I go and propose something to my boss I always end up listening to what he has to say and agreeing with him. My proposal is always left hanging in the air."

When I heard this, I asked him,

"When you talk to your boss, do you always sit facing his right side?"

"Yes" he replied.

I then told him about the polarity of the body and the fact that energy comes out of the right side and comes in from the left. I advised him that next time he went to propose something, he should sit facing the left-hand side of his boss and offer his proposal while staring at his left eye.

Later on I received news from him saying that for the first time, his boss had agreed with his proposal.

This works the other way. If you do not want to be influenced by another person's way of thinking, you should close the left side of your body up.

This technique once got me out of a tricky situation. It was an experience I will never forget.

It happened on my second visit to India. I had just got the taxi from the airport and was on the way to a railway station. Suddenly the car stopped and a companion of the driver got into the passenger side of the car. This young Indian man was large and well built. I asked the driver why it was necessary for this man to get into the car but he just said "no problem" and didn't answer my question. The car carried on going into more and more lonely territory. Seeing a little railway station coming up, I asked the driver to let me off in front of it. He looked a bit reluctant, as if to say he hadn't got to the destination yet, but consented.

The car stopped and the taxi driver asked for seventy rupees. I put together seven ten rupee notes and handed them to him from the back seat. He turned around, took the notes and counting them in front of me, he said "there are only five notes here. I need another twenty rupees." The man in the passenger seat also turned around and told me in a threatening manner to "pay twenty rupees more."

The driver, with the deft hand of a magician had removed two notes right in front of my eyes. I looked on in disbelief. I stared into his bloodshot left eye and in my mind I prayed "O infinite energy of the Universe! Please help! This man is trying to cheat me."

All was silent for a brief moment. Suddenly the driver started to shake as if he was having a fit. Seizing this opportunity to leave, I took my luggage, opened the door discreetly and got out.

The man in the passenger seat must have been scared stiff from seeing what had happened to his friend, as even though I had started to walk towards the station, he didn't move a muscle.

Afterwards I gave thanks to the Great Cosmos for getting me out of trouble.

If What You Think Is Different To What You Do, Your Body Will Become Distorted

One day, businessman Mr. A came to my practice and brought along Mr. B, his business friend. Mr. A asked me to put some energy into Mr. B for aiding with his work, since he had been good to him.

Mr. B was a big stout gentleman. While I was carrying out Ki therapy on the man, I noticed that his Ki was slightly distorted in his lumbar spine.

Afterwards, there was a phone call from Mr. A.

"What did you think of Mr. B?" he asked. "He's very nice, isn't he?"

"Mm…yes I replied. 'But I sense that he's not someone to be trusted."

"No way" he declared. "That's unthinkable."

Ten months passed and I received another phone call from Mr. A.

"I was cheated by Mr. B. I had trusted him, but he betrayed me" he said, angrily and in a harsh tone. There had been some trouble regarding investment money. So my prediction had been spot on, I thought regrettably to myself.

If what you say is different to what you do, a subtle imbalance arises in the body and mind. If this continues for a long time, the body becomes distorted. This is what I had detected in Mr. B's lumbar spine.

In actual fact, we often suffer from the inability to refuse a request from others even when it is against our wishes. Say we could look into our minds when we do this; I wonder what we would see. Most probably there would be the anger you had felt from when you were given the request, and the grudge you have against the person who made the request.

That is why, deep down, if we really do not want to take up a request or feel obligated to do something, it is better to pick up the courage and refuse. Otherwise, what we think becomes different to what we say. The body will thus become distorted, and we may become ill.

Someone once said, "Stress is something which happens when the mouth opens on it's own accord and says 'yes' even though the heart is saying 'no'."

When We Talk About Our Hopes And Dreams They Become Realized In Words, Making It Hard For Them To Become Reality

There are those who often talk about their innermost desires to others. It is normally the case that these kinds of people do not see their dreams realized.

Why is this?

The reason is because expressing your hopes and desires in words is part of the realization process. Writers have their dreams realized in words. Painters have their dreams realized in their paintings.

This is why, except when you are with friends who share the same dreams as you, you should keep your dreams close to your chest as much as you can. Making your dreams known to a lot of people may bring them one step closer to being realized, but only in the world of words, not in reality.

Also, after chatting for a long time, have you ever felt that you've lost something?

In my travels, when I was on my own and witnessed something that moved me, I would keep it to myself. As a result, I feel that my experiences have been kept alive and vivid in my mind.

If, however, you go on a trip with friends and witness something impressive, you immediately try and express the experience in words with them. The more it is spoken about, the more the immediacy and freshness of the experience is lost from your mind. Say someone then cracks a bad joke about it. The experience is now tarnished: the impressive moment now just a memory.

I would ask for those who speak a lot in everyday life to look at themselves closely. You may find you are tired from speaking so much, or that you are leaving an unfavourable impression on others whose feelings you fail to read.

For those who find themselves in this category, I recommend a bout of silence.

The method is simple. Put aside a bit of time in the day where you keep a strict silence. If you try this, the results will be immediate. Stop your tendency to talk when in the midst of people, for instance, and you will find that you are relaxed and that your mind is tranquil. Furthermore, you won't get as tired as before since you aren't losing energy unnecessarily. Listening to what people have to say will make you more considerate of other people's feelings. They will no doubt think well of you in return.

Once you control your chatter and stop telling people about your innermost dreams you will find how, more and more, the things you wish for become true.

Start The Day With Positive Words
End The Day With A Clear Mind

When we get up in the morning, our minds are immediately clouded with various thoughts.

Thinking of all the things that need to be done in the day, we let out a sigh and instantly start to feel tired.

We may start to feel depressed about this or start to worry about whether or not the important things that need to be done in the day will go according to plan.

Alternatively we may feel anxious or think in a negative way about meeting a certain person and then stay in this sorry state throughout the day.

It is a vicious circle: thinking negatively creates negative waveforms which attract more negativity.

Therefore when you wake up you should start the day by saying some positive words and repeating them two or three times over.

Your mood will be different just from doing this.

For example, say things like "today I feel great" or "everything will go well in every way" first thing in the morning.

Since there are positive waveforms in positive words and negative waveforms in negative words, if you recite this sort of thing to yourself, somehow your mind will become tranquil and you will feel better. If you don't believe me, have a go yourself.

For those who worry easily, try instead to imagine things going well for yourself. If you have a worry about a particular thing, replace it with an image of that thing going well. If you make a habit of doing this, your image will become reality. You will also become healthy, since this is what happens when one stops worrying.

Now for when you go to bed. This is also an important time in the day when your feelings can be influenced.

Have you ever watched a horror film before going to bed at night and then had a nightmare? This happens because the fear you felt from watching the film is absorbed into your mind when you go to sleep. The same happens if you feel regret over what took place during the day before going to sleep. Since to regret something is to re-enact a bad experience or mistake in your head, negative thoughts end up deep in the mind. This in turn disturbs the autonomic nerve, which has an effect on your mood. You should thus try and stop feeling regret before going to bed, just as you should avoid watching horror films at night before you sleep.

The best thing one can do is to totally empty the mind, but this is obviously very difficult. It is, however, easy to imagine a beautiful scene in your mind.

A scene of a babbling brook, for example. The water is clear and the sunrays shine through to the bottom of the river where the little pebbles glint in the light. Just by imagining this sort of scene will ensure it is absorbed deep in the consciousness.

You could also use a memory of a scene you witnessed while on your travels. Your image could be, say, a blinding white snowy mountain, or a mirror-like lake. A beautiful image will put the mind at peace.

When we wake up, we should say something positive. Before going to sleep, we should first make the mind clean and pure.

If you do these two things everyday, I am sure that not only will you feel better and become healthy, but everything will start to go well for you.

If You Deny Something, Your Capacity Will Diminish

Once a London based business attaché from a large company came to my practice in ill health. We talked and I gathered that he had become ill from the stress caused by the relationship with his boss. His own position was Section Manager.

I asked him why the relationship with his boss wasn't going well.

"Whenever I propose what I think on a matter, my boss always dismisses what I say", he explained. "Recently, whenever I try to speak he says "You don't have to tell me, I already know" and doesn't even try to listen to what I have to say."

Because of the stress of this, he had become ill. He had now really had enough of working under his boss and it had come to the stage that if his boss wasn't transferred back to Japan, then he himself would have to resign.

When he was relaxed from the Ki I told him the following.

"There are an overwhelming amount of things that we human beings do not understand in the Universe. That is why, unless we are completely sure about something, we should never dismiss what a person says. If we dismiss someone without being completely sure, then we put a restriction on our capacity. We can think of this capacity as our tolerance and recognition of other people and our depth of heart. Since your boss always dismisses what you say, his capacity has diminished so that he can no longer accommodate you. A boss with only a capacity of dealing with five people can only have five people underneath him. Is it not because your boss cannot accommodate you that it has become very difficult for you to keep hanging on and working under him?"

When I had finished speaking, it seemed that something had suddenly clicked in his mind.

"All along I have been doing the same thing as my boss" he said.

He was talking about the ten people who were working underneath him. These people were a source of worry, since they were not working like he had wanted them to. Another thing that preyed on his mind was that capable people of whom he had high expectations for had left soon after entering the company.

Being busy had something to do with it, but when one of his subordinates proposed something to him, he had a habit of cutting the person off, saying "yes, I understand" and dismissing it as "nonsense."

This is what he had suddenly realized. He had been like his boss in the dismissal of his subordinates and his capacity had been reduced to the effect that his subordinates could no longer continue working underneath him. He now understood the reason why even those who were capable at the job had left.

He took on my advice henceforth and started to listen to what his subordinates had to say. Unless he was completely confident in his own point of view, he took in any suggestions and stopped being dismissive.

The next time he visited me his face looked much healthier and he had as good as recovered from his illness. This told me that his relationship with others in his company had also improved considerably.

There Is No Inherent Good And Evil In Things Themselves. It Is People Who Decide This

Essentially, there is no good or bad in an object, situation or a conclusion.

A kitchen knife, for example, is itself a neutral thing, beyond good and evil. If it is used by someone with the intention to kill, it becomes a murderous weapon. If it is used for preparing a meal, it becomes a daily utensil.

In the same way, there is no such thing as good and bad in a situation that arises, or in a conclusion to a matter.

Some time ago the following happened. A businessman was on transfer who had finished his time in London and was due to be sent back to Tokyo. It was the day before leaving and he had moved out of his rented house into a hotel.

Mr. Isamu Mochizuki

That evening I got a call from him. He had phoned me to tell me that he had lost his passport and asked me if I could tell him where it was.

"I'm not a fortune teller, nor am I psychic, so I can't tell you where your passport is", I told him. As I did so, the man started to berate himself.

"Always at a time like this I go and do something silly. I'm just not on the ball. I'm such a stupid, pathetic idiot."

"Wait a moment." I said, putting a stop to this self-belittlement. "How about thinking in this way?" I asked, and gave him the following advice.

"The fact that you lost your passport must mean that you either dropped it when you moved to the hotel, or someone stole it off you. Either way, this is neither a good or a bad thing. You have merely taken a negative standpoint, which is why you blame yourself. Maybe the reason you can't find your passport is because you shouldn't be getting on that flight tomorrow. It might be that the plane will crash, or something bad will happen."

"I suppose if I think like that I should be grateful that I lost my passport" the Japanese businessman said.

Finally I said to him, "Try to always think of things in a positive light like I did just then. If you do, a better way will open up before you."

Ten days after this I received a letter from him. I learnt that he had managed to get his passport re-issued from the Japanese Embassy a few days after he lost it and that he had arrived safely back in Japan.

The Power Of Life

I also learnt from the letter that during the extra days he subsequently had to stay in London, he had bumped into someone from his student days. He looked at this as the reason why he had lost his passport and had his leaving date postponed.

When he and his friend started talking to each other again for the first time in twenty years, they found out that they were in the same line of work as each other, and believe it or not, they even got so far as to make business negotiations together.

He finished the letter by stating how grateful he was that he had lost his passport.

I am sure that giving him just one positive reason as to why he may have lost his passport was enough to create a very favourable outcome for him.

Chapter 6: Life And The Self

On Freedom

I cannot bear to be restricted or to have my freedom taken away from me. Since I myself am like this, I will never willingly impose restrictions or take freedom away from anyone else.

Small children are like this too. From time to time I see children who, when forced to do something by their mothers, screw up their eyes, cover up their ears with their hands and shake their heads in an attempt to close up their five senses. Even small children cannot bear to be restricted.

When I see this happen with children it makes me realize that deep down, human beings wish to be free.

In fact, although it is important for human beings to be equal, it is more important that they be free. Communist states which tried to make equality a reality found they couldn't do so while undermining the freedom of the people.

No doubt those people who undertake hard spiritual training do so because they wish to be undone from their worldly shackles and long to be in a state of inner freedom.

The following is a story I once heard about a person and his inner freedom.

There was once a young man who went to a Himalayan temple to practice meditation. All he had in his tiny room was a toothbrush and a bucket of water with which he did his daily tasks, all from washing his face to going to the toilet. There was only one meal a day, seating was on the floor, and all that could be seen of the outside was blue sky and mountains from his small window.

After his training, this young man went back to the city. He had lived a punishingly spartan life up to that point which must have felt restrictive, but being in the city again, the young man understood how city life lacked the freedom that was in fact abundant in the life in the mountains.

Here is another story about an old lady in her late eighties who used to come to my place once every few months. The old lady had been weakened in both body and mind after her husband, with whom she had been together for most of her life, had died. When she gradually regained her strength back, she said, "I never imagined freedom was such a fantastic thing."

According to the old lady, as she had married in her teens and was continually surrounded by her in-laws, she hadn't had the freedom to do what she wanted.

When her husband died she was able for the first time to get up and eat breakfast whenever she wanted to without having to worry about anyone else. When the weather was fine, she would have a walk in the garden. When it was bad, she would pass the time indoors reading a book, as in the Japanese saying 'ploughing on a fine day, reading on a rainy day'.

"You seem to be passing your days in a 'natural state of living', the ideal way of living as taught by the Chinese philosopher Laotse" I mentioned to her.

"At the moment I feel very happy and free", said the old lady. "It's just that recently the children have been visiting a lot, and they keep on bugging me about things."

"Mother, are you getting up all right? Are you eating your breakfast all right?" the children would ask, so incessantly that she would lose her patience. Being thus aggravated, on the back of the previous year's calendar she had written 'A declaration of war' and on it was a list of strict conditions for them to obey.

"Firstly, I will get up when I please and will not be criticized for it. Secondly, I will sleep when it pleases me, and will not be criticized for it. Thirdly, I will eat when I want to and will not be criticized for it", and so on, listing ten treatises in total. She laughed as she told me this.

Several years after this, the old lady passed away peacefully while having an afternoon nap on the sofa, a natural death after a natural way of living. When I heard the news from her family, I envied her.

Recently, my own mother's death has made me think deeply about the importance of freedom. For the first time, it has prompted me to feel just how lucky I was to have a mother who never pulled me back but always let me to do what I wanted. As the days pass, I feel this more strongly than ever.

"Be free in whatever you do!"

If there is one thing that God demands of us, it must be this.

The Importance Of Deciding Things Yourself

I recall an occasion when a woman who had lost her self-confidence came to my practice for healing. She was in very poor health, and looked like she was in distress. We talked over various issues, and she explained to me how she didn't feel that she was actually living her life.

By speaking to her further I realized why this was. Whenever she needed to make a decision on something she always relied on a tarot card reader, fortune-teller or clairvoyant. It wouldn't be so bad if she took their advice just as a reference, but she wasn't like that. Their opinions on matters became her opinion on matters.

When this takes place, it means that someone else, not you, is living your life. The more this kind of thing happens, the less you will feel you are living your life.

It is important that we do not leave our minds bare to others because the mind is invaluable; it is our own identity, the proof of the existence of self.

Whatever the issue is that affects you, it is you who should have the final say on it. This is important because even if you make the wrong decision, it is you who has made it, meaning it is thus you who is living your life. The feeling of being aware of living in the present should be proof of that.

If you choose to look at the long run of things, then perhaps there isn't such a thing as a wrong decision.

Taking route A, for instance, will give you a certain set of experiences. If this path isn't right for you, then you can change to route B.

If afterwards you realize that this was a mistake, then think of it as an important lesson. Making this mistake has made you who you are now. Perhaps one day you will be able to look back and be glad that you made the mistake.

No doubt when that time comes, you will cease to think of it as a mistake.

Being Critical Of Yourself Can Bring About Unexpected Repercussions

There are times when the impression you get of someone when speaking to them on the phone is totally different from when you speak to them face to face.

I once had a call from a woman who sounded to me very arrogant on the phone. When I met her however, she seemed very different.

Since I had thought her to be haughty and rude on the phone, I had begun to feel a sense of animosity towards her.

When she was standing there in front of me, however, she didn't seem arrogant at all. In fact she appeared weak and timid.

I wondered how this could be, so I was interested to talk to her to see if I could find out. She was unusually dismissive about herself and lacked confidence in the way she spoke. She was depressed from being bullied by people at work and blamed herself for it.

What I realized while speaking to her was that it was her own hatred and dismissive attitude towards herself which appeared to me as arrogance and which prompted a tide of resentment towards her to rise up from within me. From this observation, I came to the following conclusion.

From the outside, human beings are all separated as individuals, but deep down in the mind we are all connected as one. That is why if we hate ourselves and lose all self-confidence, the company we are with will also feel despised or looked down upon by us and as a result would feel resentment towards us.

In this way, by being critical and hateful towards herself, this woman had unconsciously given the impression to others that she was unpleasant, rude and arrogant and as a result, invited feelings of resentment towards her.

On the other hand, people who think kindly of themselves and are confident will leave a good impression on others and will give off a sense of modesty in both action and speech. When the mind treats the self with respect, it is transmitted directly to the person you are in contact with. This person will also feel as a result that he/she is being treated with respect. This is why those who have an inner confidence are well respected by those around them.

Those like the woman who worry that they don't seem to be getting on well with the people around them should, without delay, stop putting the blame on others.

By doing this I would like those concerned to see how other people's perceptions towards them change according to their own attitude.

If you try and change the people around you, you will only come up against resistance. If you change yourself, however, others will change with you.

Essentially, Human Beings Have No Fixed Self

Many people who see me for treatment come burdened with problems. When I discuss their problems with them, they tell me that they are in an awful mess and that nothing can be done about it.

Let's stop there and think about this.

Who is it that decides they are in an irresolvable mess?

It is the 'self'.

So what is this 'self'?

This is a difficult question to answer.

Some people may automatically say their own name. There are no doubt others who will think it is their body.

If you think about it for a while, though, the 'self' is the thing that is thinking right now. The thing that is feeling and sensing now, and the thing that is imagining something now. If you think that you are in an inescapable awful mess, then you will find yourself in such a situation. If you think "this is fun", then you will have fun. Similarly, if you think in your mind that you are suffering, then you will suffer.

From this we can gather that in order to liberate ourselves from being in a mess, we must change the way we think and feel. The question is what 'self' we decide to choose. Choosing to think in a positive way will lead us to become positive and cheerful. Choosing to think in a negative way will lead us to become negative and gloomy.

Human beings, in other words, do not have an unchanging 'self'.

Therefore, if there is an ideal state of 'self' that you wish to be in, all you have to do is choose that 'self'.

If You Try Something, No Matter How Small, A Path Will Open Up Before You

One day a Japanese student came to see me at my practice. He was in his twenties, and was studying at London University.

He had started to suffer from anxiety attacks, and had gone to hospital, but the drugs they gave him did not seem to improve his condition. Hearing about me through a friend, he came to see me. I asked him how he was feeling. He told me he could hardly ever get to sleep at night, and that when he got anxious it became difficult to breathe.

I then commenced with the Ki therapy. After a while, he said that the area around the stomach had become painful. This was a sign that it had hardened from excessive stress and anxiety but had now loosened. Around the stomach is the solar plexus which controls the autonomic nervous system. If this relaxes, it shows that the balance of the body has improved.

After a short while, he told me that the pain had gone. Suddenly, his breathing improved from shallow breaths to deep breaths from the stomach. Whilst breathing like this he fell into a deep sleep.

When he awoke from his sleep he looked refreshed. "I haven't slept this well for a while", he said, happily.

"How is University going?" I asked him.

"I go to my lectures, but I still haven't the faintest idea of what I want to do in the future" he replied.

"Isn't there something you would like to do?" I asked.

"Mmm. Not that I can think of" he replied.

"There must be something. It doesn't matter how trivial it is, have a think."

The Power Of Life

"Well, now you ask, I suppose it is having a drink with my friends in the izakaya (a kind of Japanese pub) in front of the railway station in my hometown."

"There, you see, there is something you want to do."

I recommended the young man that he go and do this. He looked surprised as if to say, "What, even something as insignificant as this?" and laughed.

"Well this I can do. In the summer I think I'll go back to my hometown. It'll be three years since I've been."

At the end of September of that year I received a phone call from him.

His voice was bright and cheerful. He had, in the end, gone back to his hometown for the first time in three years, and had spent an enjoyable time at an izakaya, having a drink with friends.

He got an idea from talking to his friends as to what he wanted to do, which was to stay at university for one more year. Unfortunately, he didn't have the funds to pay for the tuition.

He then, for the first time, looked at the possibility of applying for a scholarship and submitted an essay that was part of the criteria. To his surprise, the essay was marked very highly, and he got the scholarship.

"I was able to receive a substantial amount of scholarship money. Now I can study again next year and not worry about the fees. I'm going to do my best," he said, sounding very happy.

He graduated from university and now has a job in London which he enjoys.

From watching the progress of this university student I now firmly believe that the door is always open for one to proceed through. Whether you do or not is up to you.

Look With Your Own Eyes!
Think With Your Own Head!
Live Your Own Life!

After around two hundred and sixty years of Tokugawan Shōgunate rule, the modern-age Japanese people struggled to find a suitable new way of living.

This is because up till then, people merely obeyed orders from above; there was no room for individuality. When the Tokugawan Shōgunate ended, many people, after a life of being repressed, were in need of a new way of living where they would make decisions for themselves.

Those at the forefront of Japan's modern age, Sōseki Natsume, Shiki Masaoka, Akiko Yosano and others feared that just taking in European and American culture would not get the Japanese anywhere. They believed that if the Japanese didn't find a new way of living by themselves, then there was no way things would change for the better.

These three therein agreed that the appropriate way that people should live was according to these three precepts: 'Look with you own eyes, think with your own head and live your own life.'

In Japan, when someone sounds impressive, there is a tendency for people to agree with that person. Agreeing with the general mood may be more convenient than thinking for oneself, but in doing so you are giving up on yourself. There are many of those who have in this way given up on themselves. We can see this from looking at unscrupulous psychic trades where there is a never-ending flow of customers, and from the thriving trades of fortune telling and crystal ball gazing.

The reason why modern day Japanese care so much about other people's opinions and are therefore not so good at living their own lives may originate in the fact that deep down they still can't get over the fact that they are no longer being controlled like they were in the Tokugawa period.

The way of living as recommended by the three representatives of the Japanese modern era should be taken to heart by those modern day Japanese who still find it difficult to live their own lives.

We Should Not Put So Much Importance On Form

What actually is form?

Form, as can be seen in Martial Arts, Performing Arts or Sports, is a standard set of rules.

Because we put undue importance on the standard set of rules, we can't help but be particular about the form. Let's pursue this by looking at how people long ago thought about form.

'Shu' (to keep), 'Ha' (to break from) and 'Ri' (to take off), are teachings transmitted from long ago. The meaning of 'Shu' is to stick faithfully to the basic form set by your teacher and to learn it well. Teachings where the body is used always start with 'Shu'.

When, after constant practice, you have learnt the form well, you change it a little to adapt to your body. Keeping the basic structure the same, you remodel parts of it to make it as easy to do as possible. This is 'Ha'. You then become creative, and develop the already remodeled form further. This creatively conceived form is different from any form until now, including that of the teacher. It is your own unique form. This is 'Ri'.

In Shodō (Japanese calligraphy) these three steps are 'Kaisho (standard/printed style)', 'Gyōusho (semi-standard/semi-cursive style)' and 'Sōusho (cursive/grass style)'. Although Martial artists or Ki practitioners all teach different forms unique to them, once the form is learnt, it must ultimately be discarded. If you are concerned with keeping to the form, you will not have achieved real progress. Only once you stop being concerned with the form will you be introduced to the expanse of the inner self, and be able to stand at the entrance of a different dimensional world.

Freeing Yourself From Rules and Preferences Will Make It Easier To Live

If you are trapped by rules or preferences which say you must do things in a certain way, life becomes dull and hard. Look at how you yourself live. With the various rules and preferences that you have, do you not feel bound down by life? If you could live without these various rules and preferences, think how free your mind would be.

With this in mind, if we look closely at nature there are many things we can learn.

Let's look at water, for example.

Water is a liquid, so will fit any container. Water can also become a gas through evaporation. That means it can flow freely into even the tightest spots. However when water goes below freezing point it solidifies, becoming ice. When it becomes ice, it obeys the restrictions that govern a solid.

If we take this as a metaphor for your mind, the more you let restrictions govern you, the more your mind will change from water to ice. Your mind will only be able to receive things that are the same shape as the ice (in other words the things your preferences permit), socializing with other people will become difficult and it will become harder and harder to make your way in life.

On the other hand, if you totally release yourself from your rules and preferences and everything that restricts you, then your mind will change from water to gas. You will be in a state where there is no attachment to any particular thought, where you will be able to adapt with great flexibility to any given situation and life will become all the more enjoyable as a result.

Nature teaches us that being free depends entirely on how you conduct your mind.

All Answers Can Be Found Inside Yourself

When we are faced with a problem in our daily lives, we seek outside ourselves for the solution, be it from books, from a more experienced person, or even from a fortune-teller. If we seek outside ourselves for the answer it is very rare that we will find a solution that will truly satisfy us.

However, if you become quiet, look inside and face your inner self, you will be able to find the answer you have been searching for.

When I was young, I went on a long journey that lasted many years. When I think about it now, it was because subconsciously I was searching for something. It is like the story of the young man who went on a journey to search for the blue bird, but gave up after a while and went back home, only to find that the blue bird had been there all along. I also found what I had been looking for after I stopped travelling and faced my inner self.

A little while after my travels I started working for a company but I grew more and more tired of this way of living. During that time I had started to practise yoga. Everyday in the middle of the night, while I was doing meditation I would pray to myself, saying, "Please let me have a job that suits me best." After this I would add "If possible, a job where I can work on my own without having to commute."

From practicing this everyday, my wish did indeed come true.

I would therefore advise those who don't know what to do to find some quiet time once a day where you can reveal your problems and aspirations to yourself. If you do this, you will receive an answer.

For those who find it difficult with problems that arise in daily life, I would advise you to stop worrying. Once you have done this you must make yourself quiet and tell yourself "This problem has been completely resolved, thank you so much", and then wait for the solution to arrive.

If you carry this out, the answer may come to you either as a feeling you get, it might alternatively spring up from the print in a magazine you happen to be reading, or it may come from something said in a conversation with a friend.

In any case, if you are stuck with a problem, try this method.

1. First you must stop your worrying.
2. Quieten your mind then confide the problem you face with your inner self.
3. Say "this problem has been completely resolved" and then "thank you."
4. Be mindful that the answer may be given to you at any point in your daily life and just wait for this to happen.

If you really want to be happy, first of all you must imagine and believe in it yourself. Real happiness can, after all, only be found in your own heart.

We put a lot of effort into looking for happiness because most of us believe that happiness is found outside ourselves. This is why most people think they will only be happy if they have their own house, a new car, a beautiful looking partner or designer bags and clothes. They believe that they will become happy once their desires are fulfilled. In other words, because you do not have these various things that you want you are unhappy, and this belief that you are lacking in things takes over the mind. Even when you think you have become happy, this belief goes on creating an even greater desire.

Even if you live in a five million pound mansion, if you don't feel happiness in your heart then you are not happy.

However, if your heart is filled with peace and happiness then you are happy, regardless of the surroundings you are in. If it rains, then appreciate what it brings. If it turns sunny, well that is good also. If you think like this you will appreciate everything.

Therefore, no matter how awful a situation you find yourself in, find a bit of time when you are on your own where it is silent and say to yourself "At this moment I am at peace, and happy" and repeat this everyday. If you do this, your mind will be filled with the belief that you are at peace and are happy. Before long, the waveforms emitted from your belief will be acted upon by the Universe and you will become as spiritually and materially happy as you have ever been.

Not Having Money Can Be Tough, But On The Other Hand, Having Too Much Can Bring Suffering

In this modern society we live in, it is tough if you don't have any money, but having too much can bring with it problems, for money too has the power to take freedom away from people.

I heard from somewhere that the biggest worry of Mr. Rockerfeller, one of the richest people in the world, was not knowing what kind of figure his entire wealth amassed to. It may be a hard thing for ordinary people like us to understand, but maybe we can think of it in the following way.

Imagine having a painting by Van Gogh that is worth tens of millions of pounds in your house. You would be too scared to leave your house unattended. You may start to get pains in your stomach from the worry.

Even though we know that having money can bring with it suffering in this way, we cannot help but be attached to it.

There are also people who become ill because of their attachment to money. Quite often, there are wealthy people who come to my practice, afflicted with an illness but unable to explain the cause of it. They have been diagnosed with a particular illness even though on appearance, they do not look ill. I think that because they have money in various different banks, they become highly strung from the worry, which causes an imbalance in the body and makes them ill as a result. I suppose you can tell because after I give them Ki treatment, most of them instantly loosen up and relax from their state of high tension. Unfortunately though it gets a lot worse than this. There are those who cannot go on living because of receiving a large amount of money.

I once heard about an elderly Muslim man, who hit the ten million pound jackpot in the lottery with the first ticket he ever bought. He had been living a simple life as a public toilet cleaner, and would have been very happy just to have won a couple of hundred pounds, but as the amount he won was so ridiculously large, he was at a loss as to what to do with it. He went and saw the Imam at his local mosque and told him that he wished to donate all the money to them but was told his dirty money was not wanted. Therefore this pious elderly Muslim, not knowing what to do with the money, committed suicide.

After hearing stories like this, I believe that the best way is to have just the amount of money that you need, and to keep your account topped up with the same amount that you spend, without being tempted to add any more.

Chapter 7: Life And Living

About 'En' (The Bond Between People)

As someone who has never needed to advertise for my Ki therapy practice and Yoga class, I would describe 'en' as the amazing and mysterious connection that exists between people.

There is a saying in Japan, "sode furiaumo tashō no en" ("even a brush of the sleeve is a small 'en'"). In the Japanese Kōjien dictionary it is explained as, "Even brushing the sleeve of a stranger is from the 'en' of your past life. In other words, even the smallest event is the result of your 'en'."

If this is the case, then those who come to my Yoga class and Ki clinic must therefore have an especially strong 'en' with me.

Curiously enough, there are also those who are rarely able to come or cannot come at all even though they try to. These people I presume either have very weak 'en' or no 'en' with me.

There was once a man who, several times a year, suffered from a slipped disc in his back. Every time it occurred he found it very hard to bear, and was forced to take a number of days off from work. One day he heard from a colleague at work that there was someone who could mend his back in just one session. He asked for the address, and found out to his surprise that it was the house just diagonally opposite from his own. He immediately went to this house (my house) and fortunately his back was healed after one session. By that time, however, his transfer back to Tokyo had been arranged. He lamented over the fact that had he come to my place sooner, he would not have had to endure years of physical pain. It could be said, therefore, from this respect, that his 'en' with me was weak.

Another story concerns a woman who booked an appointment to see me over the phone. During our telephone conversation, I had a feeling she would get lost trying to find my place. I therefore gave her very clear directions to my house and was confident she couldn't go wrong. However, on the day of the appointment, there was no sign of her when her time came. Finally, after the next person had arrived for his session, there was a phone call from her. Apparently she had got off by mistake at an Underground station on a different line with a similar name to the one nearest my house. My directions would therefore have made no sense to her. She was exhausted, so I proposed that she call me and book an appointment again when it was more convenient for her. I never heard from her again. Maybe there was no 'en' between this lady and I.

On the other hand, there are also those like this.

This is a story of a woman who came from outside London by train to have therapy at my practice. When she arrived at Victoria Station (in London), she realized that she had forgotten her address book in which she had written my telephone number and address at home. The moment she realized her misfortune, a middle-aged Japanese lady passed in front of her. Automatically, she told her my name, and asked if by any chance she might know my address. By a stroke of luck, this lady was one of my Yoga students. By another stroke of luck, she happened to live just one stop from my house on the Underground. Very kindly, she offered to take this woman, who had no knowledge of London to the door of my house. When I saw this woman being dropped off at the entrance of my house, I realized that her 'en' with me was strong.

Those at my Yoga class also keenly feel the existence of 'en'.

Many people tell me that they feel a closeness with people they meet for the first time at the class, as though they have known them for a long time.

Once at my Yoga class, the following reunion also happened.

A man had been transferred by his company to England from Japan. He had married once in Japan but had divorced and re-married again and now had a child. By chance, he happened to bump into his ex-wife at my yoga class. She was now living in England, having married an Englishman. They looked at each other for a while, slightly bewildered as if to say "what are you doing here?" Afterwards, because of this chance meeting, they were able to clear the ill feeling between them that had remained since they had parted.

Every time I witness or hear about these sorts of occurrences, I am reminded of the mysterious nature of 'en' and I feel more and more that if we respect the 'en' of other people, then our lives will benefit as a result.

If You Don't Want To Feel Failure, Don't Expect

Often in our daily lives we either consciously or unconsciously do things while expecting something in return.

For example, when you give a present to someone, or do something for someone, do you not expect something in return from that person? Sometimes we grumble to ourselves, thinking, "after all I did for him, he doesn't do anything in return", or "what kind of attitude is that? He should be grateful for what I did for him." There are even times when we fall out with someone because of the expectations we have.

When our expectations are not met, we feel failure. That is why when you give things to or do things for someone it is better not to expect a single thing in return. If you do then receive something from that person, you will be overjoyed all the more since it is something you hadn't expected. In this way you will not fall out with anyone. It is better not to expect anything from your friends, children or partner. From not having any expectations, you will not be disappointed by them. This is one of the ways in ensuring long lasting relationships.

"If you don't want to be disappointed, it's best not to expect anything." When I mentioned this to a group of people, a man who was there said, "that makes a lot of sense" and proceeded to tell me about an experience of his. He told me that when he was recommended a good restaurant to eat at, he would, without delay, go out and eat there. He was, however, usually always disappointed with the food. On the other hand, when he ate at a restaurant he just happened to come across, it was often the case that he walked out happy and satisfied with his meal. "In other words" he said, "if a restaurant is recommended to me, I go to it with my own high expectations for which the dishes served in the restaurant have to live up to. I therefore end up being disappointed with the food. On the other hand, I don't have a high standard of expectation for the places I happen to chance upon, so I usually find the food surprisingly tasty."

Just as my words had made a lot of sense to him, what this man said made a lot of sense to me too.

Forgiveness

When someone does something really bad to us, we feel as if we will never be able to forgive that person but it is only a matter of time usually before we forget all about it. There are however some things that we find ourselves unable to forgive. Even though we may be persuaded to forgive by our friends, the truth of the matter is we just cannot bring ourselves to do it.

We realize how difficult forgiving can be when we imagine the feelings of those who have been the victims of terrible acts. This is because we think that to forgive the offender implies that we approve of his or her actions and it is this thought that makes us even more determined not to forgive them.

Let's look closely at the concept of forgiveness. To forgive someone does not mean you are forgetting the crime. It merely means that you are letting go of the negative feelings you have towards the person. You do not have to agree with or cancel out everything that has been done to you. All that is needed is for the negative thoughts between you and the other person to disappear. If this is all that needs to be done, surely then we should all be able to forgive.

The act of forgiving can be said to be a process for healing one's heart and mind.

The Japanese word for 'to forgive' is 'yurusu'. It is said that the word 'yurusu' originates from 'yurushi', the same origin as the verbs 'yurumu' and 'yurumeru' meaning 'to become loose' or 'to relax'.

This is why people who cannot forgive are unable to loosen themselves and therefore cannot truly relax. I mentioned this once at my Yoga class.

After class the following week, a woman who had attended the class the week before approached me to talk about herself.

"When I was listening to what you were saying the other session, I was certain that there was no one I knew whom I could not forgive. However, this last week I was checking through the people I know and I realized there is one person I still can't forgive."

"Who is that person?" I asked.

"My father," she replied.

Her father had died young when she was only a child. Because of this, deep down, she had always been unable to forgive him.

"Perhaps because of this, after I have been in a Yoga pose and lie down to relax, I always have a blocked feeling in my solar plexus area", she said.

After hearing this I gave her the following advice.

"Make an image of your father after you lie down and relax, and repeat over and over again, "I completely forgive you now Father."

After a month of doing this, the blocked feeling in her chest disappeared.

"It was really terrible when my father died," she told me. "I became fearful that if I myself had children and died early like my father, they would have to go through what I did. It was this fear and also the inability to forgive my father that was lodged deep down in my mind."

After realizing that she still had not forgiven her father, by thus forgiving him, in other words letting go of her negative feelings towards him, she was finally able to heal herself.

Later on she became pregnant and gave birth safely after a long time of being unable to conceive.

Point Out The Bad Points In Children, But Don't Criticize Them

I don't think there is a single parent who doesn't worry about their children.

After talking to many parents I realized that they all have a lot of worries on their minds. An especially common worry is that their children are not listening to what they say. This frustrates them, and they take it out on the disobedient child by pointing out his or her shortcomings. They may not actually tell the child, but they still feel critical towards them. Children are very sensitive, so if you criticize them, they will be affected. If, for example, you tell a child that they are "stupid, and good for nothing", then the child will take these words to heart, and the more these words are repeated to them, the more the child will start to believe them.

It is better, therefore, to look at the good points rather than the bad points, and openly praise the child. For example, if you say, "you have these good qualities about you, so if you try, you will succeed", then surely the child will surely be influenced positively by these words.

School sports teachers say that if you just point out the faults of a student, and try to correct them, a year will pass without much progress. On the other hand, if you point out the merits of the student and develop these good points, then in a year the student will dramatically improve. It is said that as the good points improve, the bad points become less noticeable.

When I ask those parents who worry about their children whether or not they are subconsciously critical of their children's faults, most of them reply that they are.

Someone once said that you can be critical of the child as long as you don't tell them. I disagree.

Since the parent is a person living under the same roof and even sharing the same blood, these feelings cannot fail to be picked up by the child. They detect the criticism in their parents' minds, and thus become rebellious as a result.

Those who realize that subconsciously they have been disapproving of their child's weak points should make a conscious effort to stop feeling like this. Instead, recognize the good points of the child, and praise them. If you do this, you will certainly see a distinct change in the child.

For those who believe in reincarnation, there is the theory that our children become ours because, for their own reasons, they choose us as parents. In order to have certain experiences in this life we plan a set of circumstances for this life before we are born. We exist here and now because the great power of the Universe has worked through us to make these experiences reality.

If you find yourself disapproving of your child because of their disobedience, then please try and pray in the following way.

"My son (or my daughter), we are very grateful that you chose us to be your parents. From now on I trust you will pick the best path in life."

There is a wonderful power that comes from praying. If you have time to worry about your child, then use it to pray for them.

Obstacles And Hardships Are Here To Polish The Soul

From the outside, we all look different. Once we start to think of how there are people who are beautiful, clever, and wealthy, and others who are not so, we may feel we want to speak out against the injustices of the world. However, we are all equal on a spiritual level. This is because, no matter what kind of person we are, we all possess a diamond called the soul. The only difference comes from whether this diamond is polished or looks just like a normal pebble.

When a diamond is cut and the surface polished, it will sparkle brightly. If you cut and polish many sides of the diamond, then these many sides will sparkle brightly. If you cut and polish all the sides of the diamond, then the diamond will sparkle in perfect brilliance.

Just like for the diamond, there is a necessity for us, while we are in this world, to cut and polish the elemental stone that is our soul. The things that help to cut and polish us are the obstacles and hardships that befall us in life.

When we rise above these obstacles and hardships we are able to refine the soul and make ourselves better human beings. The soul will shine with brilliance, and people will be drawn to this.

Let us look, for example, at someone who is brought up in a well-off family and is able to have anything he wants. He enjoys his life without any hardship. You may see him as being very lucky, but you wouldn't, I suspect, be inspired by his life.

On the other hand, they have been people such as Abraham Lincoln, who came from a poor home, overcame various hardships to become a lawyer and then went onto become the sixteenth President of the United States of America, using his term in office to free the black slaves, Helen Keller, who overcame her three sensory handicaps, Thomas Edison, who immersed himself in his research as an inventor and Mahatma Gandhi, who achieved India's independence from England through peaceful means. When we learn about the lives of these kinds of people we are all deeply moved.

This is because when they rose above the hardships that stood in their way, their souls were polished and shone brightly.

I myself was once a witness to a soul in its brightest state. One day, by chance, when I switched the television on, it was showing the life of the blind pianist Takeshi Kakehashi. He had come an impressive second in the world renowned Long-Thibaud International Contest, a gateway to musical success for young musicians.

Apparently, because he was totally blind, he had been rejected from every school he tried to enter.

Fortunately, the Preparatory Course of the State University of Music and Dramatic Arts in Vienna, Austria received him in spite of his blindness, and he practiced there diligently everyday. Unfortunately, however, that same year he developed a tumour on his eyeball.

He went back to Japan to have an operation to remove the tumour, and after his rehabilitation returned to Vienna to study. It is the words he said during this period that resonated within me, and which I still remember clearly.

"When I became ill, I realized that living is not something to be taken for granted. The moment now is all that matters to me. When I am engrossed in playing the piano I am truly living in the moment."

When he was twenty-one, Mr. Kakehashi applied for the Long-Thibaud International Contest.

Out of two hundred and seven applicants, he proceeded to the last six. Here, waiting for him was another big challenge to overcome. As well as a piece of music of his choice, he was instructed two months in advance to learn a modern piece of music composed especially for the competition.

It was a very long piece of music, and apparently up till that point no one had succeeded in playing it from memory. He dedicated a large amount of time reading the Braille script of the music score, and learnt the piece by heart from listening to his mother's playing of it. In this way he memorized the piece in a short time, and overcame this huge challenge.

Soon the day of the competition came. He was led onto the stage by his mother, and took his seat at the piano. The conductor signalled the start of the performance by tapping his baton on the piano, and thus the performance began. The movement of his hands was amazing to watch - no one could have guessed he was totally blind. From watching I realized that there was 'Ki' running through his fingers. Then, some time into the performance, a strange thing started to happen. Tears started to roll down the faces of the people in the audience as they listened to the music. Even the conductor had tears rolling down his face as he conducted the orchestra.

I had seen Mr. Takeshi Kakehashi's soul, having overcome various hardships, shine brilliantly and with these eyes, I can be sure, I saw the audience shed tears, deeply moved and enveloped by the aura of his soul.

When You Sympathise With Someone, Don't Let Their Grief Take You Over

Everyday on the news on TV, we see victims of various kinds of incidents. We also often hear about unfortunate things that happen to people we know. There are times when we sympathise strongly with these people. After doing this have you not also felt under the weather or become ill as a result?

To sympathise is of course no bad thing. It is in fact a perfectly natural thing to do. But when you start to worry needlessly and become unwell from the stress some action should be taken on your part to stop this from happening.

In September 2001, for example, when the multiple terrorist attacks happened in America, there were a number of people who came to my practice emotionally disturbed from the shock of seeing people jump out of the Twin Towers on TV.

Again, a man whose friend had gone to the dentist to have a wisdom tooth removed told me this story.

During the operation the anaesthetic did not work completely and his friend had to go through a terrible amount of pain. His company of around ten or so friends listened intently as he recounted his story, and fully empathized with him. He related his account realistically and in as much detail as possible in order to convey to them exactly the ordeal he went through.

When he finally finished recounting the event, his friends went back to their homes, and that night, all those who had listened to the story suffered from toothache.

Here is another experience of a woman who came to my practice for treatment. Her chest felt tight, and her head felt so heavy that she was having trouble just holding it up.

This had happened recently when her neighbour, who had lost her husband, came round to see her. She sympathized with the widow and listened to her story for five hours non-stop. Halfway through the story, as she empathized with her neighbour's suffering, her chest gradually became uncomfortably tight. Even a week later, her chest was tight and breathing still difficult and she was having trouble sleeping at night.

From these stories we can see that while it is fine that we sympathize with others, we must not let ourselves be taken over by the distress the other person feels. We must be attentive to how our body is reacting as we listen and sympathize with another person's woes. Then once we detect a sign that our body is reacting against the other person and their story, without being rude we must change the tone of the conversation to a more cheerful one. Otherwise, we should end the conversation by saying something like "sorry, I don't have much time right now, let's talk about it later."

The important thing to remember when you are sympathizing with what someone is saying is to consciously choose to be happy and cheerful, because when we sympathize with someone we subconsciously tend to choose to be anxious, self-indulgently sad and gloomy.

How To Make A Friendship Last Long

I believe a long-lasting relationship with a true friend is rare and difficult to achieve and I doubt I am alone in thinking that.

Even a childhood friend who you meet again when you are adults may be distant and indifferent, with none of the innocent playfulness of before. Perhaps this is because we start to think of our social standing and what each of us has to offer the other.

I think it is rare for someone to have a couple of friends, or even just one friend who leaves all of this out of consideration.

The Power Of Life

The majority of us, including myself, may have to admit that we do not have friends like this.

Some people end their friendship with someone after just a minor quarrel. I often hear from people who tell me that they have lost contact with a close friend with whom they had previously been inseparable.

There are also those who cannot patch things up with a friend, since they cannot forgive them for what they said when they had an argument as if the friend had walked over their clean carpet with muddy shoes.

Apparently, the main reason to why this happens is because you get too close to your friend, and start to interfere in their matters.

People long ago had the same type of relationships with one another as we do today.

It's likely that they also pondered over how a close relationship with a friend could be maintained.

About two thousand three hundred years ago, the Chinese philosopher Sōshi said these words.

"The watery wise man sees his friendship deepen. The sugary simpleton sees his friendship disappear."

In other words, the wise man makes friends with someone calmly and simply as if like water and gains from doing so a deep friendship, whereas the simpleton makes friends with someone thickly and intensely like amazake (a thick, sweet Japanese alcoholic drink) and has his friendship cut short quickly.

If the food you eat everyday suddenly became very rich in taste, what would you do? You would quickly get sick of eating it and would not want to eat it every day.

Similarly, how about if the water you drink every day became sweet like amazake? You would quickly tire of the sickly sweetness in your mouth. Water is simple and tasteless, so we cannot get sick of it even if we drink it everyday, continuously for decades. It will always be able to quench our thirst.

Sōshi says that the key to keeping a true friendship with someone for long is to be calm and simple like water. It seems there is a need to listen to the wisdom of our ancestors who lived two thousand three hundred years ago.

When Frightened In The Midst Of Darkness, People Seek The Maternal Spirit

I was in my twenties. During this time, I had been living in London for a while, attending a language school as well as working part-time.

My part time job involved the delivery of documents from a company to various other offices of different companies in the City from the evening on. One day, I was delivering documents that were requested by an office on one of the higher floors of a very tall building. This office must have been on the fortieth floor or there abouts. From this floor, there was a panoramic view of London. Normally this building would be full of businessmen, but when I was there, being after work hours, it was quiet.

After handing over the business papers, I went into the lift (alone) and pressed the button for the Ground floor. I felt the lift accelerate down. Suddenly, it began to plummet like an object in freefall. First I felt a strange sensation like my body was floating in mid-air, then I fell down to the ground with a thud. I felt a huge force pull me down to the floor of the lift. With the shock of this force, I passed out unconscious on the ground.

When I came to my senses, the lift had come to a standstill. In a panic I stood up and looked at the light showing the floor number. I realized then that I had not yet reached the ground floor but had stopped on the way down.

I banged the door and shouted for help, but in the silence no one answered my pleas. While I looked around for a phone or a means to contact the people in the building, the lights suddenly went out. Everything went pitch black. I rubbed my eyes and stretched them wide open, but in the heavy blackness I could not detect any trace of illumination.

I was trapped in this dark, confined space. After a while, through the gap in the lift, a warm breeze carried with it the smell of machine oil.

Overwhelmed with the fear of the dark and the fear of being crushed in this narrow space, I struggled to breathe. I banged on the door and shouted for help. Still not a stir. The minutes ticked by. My fear and anxiety grew by the moment.

This was the first time in my life that I had experienced a feeling of claustrophobia and a real fear of the dark.

I felt more and more helpless and despondent and like a soldier in battle at the moment of death I was at the point of calling out for my mother. Just then, two guards came at long last from the lower floors to come and save me. They prized the lift doors open, and freed me from the darkness. I had been confined for a total of about thirty minutes, but it felt more like several hours.

The fear I had felt carried on for days. For a short while I was scared of getting into a lift and even had nightmares about it. Even now, I still remember that feeling of fear, and for a long time afterwards I asked myself why I felt compelled to shout for my mother.

According to the people who fought in the War in the Pacific, soldiers who were on the point of death on the battlefield would call out for their mothers before dying.

This is I believe because people prefer a God with the female characteristics of mercy and calm tolerance to a God with the male characteristics of strict rational justice. It is also, I believe because people in actual fact long for Mother Nature, the Virgin Mary and Mother Universe, through their own mother in this world.

In most Catholic countries, the worship of the Virgin Mary is said to be even more popular than for Jesus Christ.

Nearly thirty years on from this experience of being overcome with fear in that dark, confined space, I realize now that at that time I subconsciously longed for the Cosmic Universal mother (the Divine Maternity) through my mother in this world.

Chapter 8: Life And Yoga

What Is Yoga?

It is said that the origin of the word 'Yoga' is the Sanskrit word 'Yuj' meaning 'to join', as in to join a horse and cart.

Yoga practice focuses on three things: body, breathing and meditation. You can learn about the whole practice in 'the Yoga Sutras'. The author of the Sutras is a man called Patanjali, who lived in the second century BC.

Patanjali defines Yoga as 'a way to calm the agitation of the mind'. For this to work, there are eight levels in the Yoga Sutras that need to be mastered.

These eight levels also correspond to a first, a middle and a last stage, the goal being 'Kaivalya', an absolute state of oneness.

The first stage consists of two levels, 'Yama' and 'Niyama'.

The first level 'Yama' translates as 'admonishment'. This is a moral admonishment, which says we shouldn't do bad things, since if we do it will prey on our conscience and become an obstacle to meditation.

The second level, 'Niyama' is a set of religious criteria and translates as 'encouragement to do good things'.

Next is the middle stage which consists of Asanas, Pranayama and Pratyahara.

The third level, Asanas, is a set of teachings concerning the body. It shows us how we can sit for thirty minutes or an hour in a good posture, without any discomfort in the body. Just by doing Asanas you can make yourself healthy, and make any irregularities in the body disappear. This is why nowadays many Yoga practices just teach Asanas.

The fourth level, Pranayama, is a method for breathing and also translates as 'controlled breathing'. Doing this breathing method stops irregular, shallow breathing.

The fifth level, Pratyahara, translates as 'withdrawal'. It teaches us how to withdraw the senses we use in the outside world.

The last stage consists of 'Dharana', 'Dhyana' and 'Samadhi'. The sixth level, 'Dharana', translates as 'concentration' and means the concentration of the spirit, where the mind is kept in an unchanging state.

The seventh level, 'Dhyana', translates as 'contemplation' or 'meditation'. In China, this word 'Dhyana' was changed to 'Zenna' and emerged in Buddhism, as 'Zen'.

The eighth level, 'Samadhi', translates as 'fulfillment'. This is the state of superconsciousness or enlightenment.

Finally, the goal of all these methods is 'Kaivalya', the absolute state of oneness. It may be quite a task, but if you can memorize these eight levels and their methods then you will be able to see exactly which one you are on at any given time.

Yoga Breathing

In Yoga, the breathing techniques are called 'Pranayama', which control the life energy 'Prana' and can also be translated as 'controlled breathing'.

The breathing techniques in Yoga are not just for taking in oxygen, they are also for taking in the energy which fills the entire Universe.

It is said that originally, the breathing exercises in Yoga were designed to deepen meditation. By controlling the breath the autonomic nerve is stimulated, making it easy to be controlled, and this relaxes the mind as a result.

Practicing Yoga breathing exercises before meditation will help you to meditate deeper. However, there are also many further benefits.

In Yoga, breathing is done through the nose, and not through the mouth, except for a few special cases. Breathing through the nose with the mouth closed is practised until it becomes natural. For a newcomer this may seem trivial, but in order to maintain good health it is actually extremely important. When breathing through the nose, the dust in the air is caught by the hairs in the nostrils and the finer particles are trapped by the nose membrane. The air is then warmed up in the nasal passage where it attains the appropriate humidity and finally flows into the lungs.

However, when we breathe through the mouth, dust and cold dry air is inhaled directly, and this harms the throat and the lungs. Most young people nowadays suffer from ill health because they breathe through their mouths.

Furthermore, breathing techniques stimulate and thus reinvigorate the brain. This is especially so in the various Yoga techniques in which the right and left nostrils are used in turn. When air is slowly inhaled using one nostril only, it stimulates the nerve that controls the sense of smell. Since this nerve is directly connected to the brain, the brain is stimulated as a result.

In this way, breathing techniques prevent senility. I have heard it is a proven fact that people who practice the art of 'kōdō' (the art of incense smelling) do not become senile. This is probably because, by smelling, they are stimulating the nerve that controls the sense of smell and are therefore also stimulating the brain.

In the breathing technique described above where the nostrils are used in turn to inhale and exhale, breathing with the right nostril causes the mind to look outside of itself and breathing with the left nostril causes the mind to look inside of itself. Thus, by practicing this breathing exercise, the mind becomes balanced and as a result, depression can be prevented or alleviated.

Furthermore, with practice of these Yoga breathing exercises, you will become energized. This is because since you are breathing with your diaphragm, your lungs are filled right to the bottom with oxygen. It is said that the area of lungs used when breathing with the chest is thirty jō (a counter for the Japanese tatami mat - one jō has a dimension of approximately six feet by three feet), but that when breathing with the stomach this increases to sixty jō.

From this we can see just how much more effective it is to breath from the diaphragm. The oxygen that fills up to the bottom of the lungs is transferred to all sixty trillion molecules that make up the body, energizing each one of them and making them work more vigorously. Collectively, they combine to create a body that is resistant to cancer and other illnesses.

This is gradually being recognized by medical institutions and doctors are also beginning to teach how breathing techniques can boost the immune system and be a prevention to illnesses. My Yoga students also tell me that they have read doctors comments in London magazines on how breathing exercises can prevent diseases of the brain.

Yoga Poses

The series of movements which form the Yoga poses are called Asanas.

When the body is stretched, bent backwards, curved and twisted, the flow of Ki called 'Prana' (life energy) runs along the 'Nadi'(Chinese meridian and Prana pathway).

However, just practicing Asanas as mere stretching or physical exercises will not stimulate the flow of Ki in the body. Those who do Yoga with this intention will not improve their health. I understood this after practising Yoga Asanas and trying out different techniques with people who were suffering from an illness. I realized that great benefit can be got from following these four points:

Firstly, the movements must be done slowly. Do not speed up.

Secondly, match your breathing with your movements. For example, breathe out slowly as you bend your body forwards. By the time you have finished moving, you should have breathed out all you can. Similarly when breathing in, you should have breathed in all you can by the time you have finished moving.

Thirdly, when you have finished the movement and are in the pose, you should concentrate on the places in the body that are painful. If you do this, the pain will occupy the cells of the brain. When this happens, any distracting thoughts in the mind will disappear. When you concentrate on pain, you can put a stop to anxieties about work and other matters.

Fourthly, when you go back to the rest position after holding a pose, feel your muscles and joints loosen slowly back from their stretched position. This will make you naturally aware of your body, and your ability to concentrate will increase.

Please practice Asanas with these four points in mind.

The poses may look just the same from the outside even if you do not follow the four points. If you do follow them however, you will see that there is a tremendous difference in the effects.

The Key And Goal Of Asanas

When the body is curved, twisted and bent backwards in Yoga, the sympathetic nerve of the autonomic nervous system is activated. After making a pose, you must lie down facing upwards and relax. This is called the Shava-asana (the corpse pose).

When the Shava-asana is practised after activating the sympathetic nerve through making a pose, the secondary sympathetic nerve is then activated to calm it down. When the secondary sympathetic nerve is activated, the body automatically loosens up. The sense of relaxation from doing this is remarkable. Many people who practice Yoga say that they are able to continue with it due to this feeling of relaxation.

It is said that doing the Shava-asana for ten minutes has the same effect as sleeping for a couple of hours.

If you are able to relax deeply, you will feel your body cling fast to the ground as though you have become one with the earth. Alternatively you may feel that your arms and legs have disappeared or that you are floating in mid-air, or feel a sense of oneness, as if your mind and body has blended with the Universe.

Previously I explained that in the word 'relax', 're' means 'again' and 'lax' means 'to loosen', and that the word 'relax' signifies being at one with the Universe.

So no matter how beautifully or perfectly you do a Yoga pose, no matter how many poses you perform or how long the poses are practised for, if the Shava-asana is not carried out at the end, you cannot say you have practised Yoga.

On the other hand, if you only do two or three poses but are able to relax deeply and comfortably you can be sure to have successfully practised Yoga.

If You Continue Practising Yoga Throughout Your Life, You Will Develop Great Power

If you try Yoga just a couple of times you will not be able to notice any difference.

Once you start Yoga, you must continue with it. In order that you will be able to continue, you must not make any impractical plans. There are people who make plans from the start to practise everyday, but when a day arises when they cannot practise they see this as a failure and give up. If there is a day or two or even a week when you cannot practise, there is always the day after that when you *can* practise. If you think in this way, you will be able to continue with Yoga.

It is fine in any case to miss a couple of days. If you are not too strict on yourself you will find that you are able to continue with it.

You must also not compare yourself with others. There are, by nature, human beings who have stiff bodies and others who have flexible ones. Yoga is different to stretching and exercise, so it does not matter if your body is stiff and your pose does not look good (refer back to the section in this chapter on Yoga poses).

There are those who start Yoga because they are ill, but give it up after regaining their health. It is often the case that these people become ill again a year after giving up Yoga, and so have to restart their practise.

Even if a person's health improves after starting Yoga, continuous practise is still needed to maintain this state of health. If Yoga is given up at this point, the illness will return. However, if you keep practising Yoga past this point you will lose your susceptibility to getting ill. Furthermore, if you continue to practice Yoga on and on you will become amazingly healthy.

If you persist with Yoga, you will reach a point when if one day you do not practise it you will feel as if something is missing or you will feel unclean, like the feeling you get when you have forgotten to brush your teeth. When this happens, you should congratulate yourself, as your body has become accustomed to Yoga. Once this is achieved, you should keep on practicing Yoga for the rest of your life. If you do, you will live long and avoid senility. In old age you will be able to do everything for yourself, and even a little for other people. In this way, you will prove yourself very useful even when you grow old.

If you carry on in this way, two days before you die, a slight sign of ageing appears, and you acknowledge that you are going to the other world. When the time is right, you tidy up your belongings, and go to bed. When the body is near to death, more endorphins are released in the brain for those who practice yoga continuously than for those who do not. These endorphins have the power to get rid of anxieties and pain and make sure that you take your leave of this world in a blissful sleep.

Please try to continue practicing Yoga all through your life.

Practice Yoga With Confidence

This can be said for everything, but when doing Yoga, it is important to practice it with confidence. The result of doing something with conviction as opposed to doing it without conviction is very different.

Say, for example you start Yoga to get over an illness. There is a huge difference in the outcome from doing it with doubts in your mind, thinking "will I really cure myself simply by doing what seems to be just a work out?" and in the outcome from doing it with conviction, thinking "if I continue practicing Yoga, my body will become more balanced, my immune system will get stronger, and I will get better."

There is a term called the 'placebo effect'. This occurs when a fake medicine (placebo) is prescribed and becomes as effective as the real medicine.

For example, say I was prescribed sugar instead of real medicine. When I put my belief in the effectiveness of what has been prescribed and my faith in the doctor who prescribed it, a 'placebo effect' acts on the sugar to make it become a remedy for the illness.

Strangely enough, even for bogus drugs like this, if taken with conviction, they will work as well as or even better than the real drugs.

If this is the effect you can get from taking fake medicine, imagine the effect you will get from practicing Yoga with a conviction that your illness will be healed.

Yoga And Food

The body is the same as a temple. A temple is a place where people undertake discipline in order to become one with the Universe. The body too occupies the same role for each one of us. The temple-body is maintained by food, so food is important in keeping the body in the best condition possible.

Yoga does not say that you have to fast, but it does recommend that you have a modest diet.

To have a modest diet is very important for the health. There are countless proverbs in many countries from long ago that warn us of the dangers of over-eating such as these which have been translated: "If you want to be healthy, stop eating before you get full" and "an eighty percent full stomach won't need a doctor." This tells us that people long ago must have known about the ill effects of over-eating. Nowadays too, it could be argued that most illnesses are caused by over-eating.

So a modest diet is good, but what is it that we should eat? Before we get to that, let's look at the make-up of human teeth.

Human beings have only two canine teeth for the top set and two for the bottom set. It therefore seems that human teeth have not been designed to be used for eating meat. Instead, there are as many as twenty molars; five on either side and on both sets. Evidently, human teeth have been designed for chewing on fruits, berries, grain and vegetables.

We can therefore denounce from this that it is only wise to make pulses and vegetables our main diet, and make meat and fish an occasional addition.

However, when there is a sudden change in our diet from what we are used to, it is bad for the body.

For example, if a Japanese person suddenly switches to a Western diet, then they may become diabetic. This is because the DNA of the Japanese, who are agricultural people, is constructed so that in case of a bad harvest, the staple food that they eat is absorbed well in the body.

This is the same the other way. If a Westerner suddenly changes to a diet of rice and vegetables, it may be bad for the stomach. I have heard that for hunting people, the intestine is made so that meat is digested well and excreted quickly and is shorter in length than the intestines of agricultural people.

It is also a possibility that your vibrations can be altered by the food you eat. For example, meat, produced by the killing of an animal, carries the vibrations of the fear the animal experienced at the time of death. For this reason, it is said that eating meat can become an obstacle to meditation.

If we are to look into the vibrations of food, we need to look at the vibrations emitted from the origins of the food, the way it has been cooked, and how it is eaten. There is a saying in Islam, 'if you are angry when you eat, your food will turn into poison'.

Similarly, eating a lot of rich and spicy food is advised against, as an obstacle to meditation.

There are many different things that people say about food, but from my experience, there is no need to go and intentionally change your diet if you practice Yoga.

A couple of months after starting Yoga any desire to drink alcohol disappeared from my mind. If I had forced myself to give up alcohol, I would still feel the urge to drink when surrounded by friends who are all drinking, but since my desire has faded naturally, this doesn't happen to me. I do enjoy a sip of beer when people make a toast, but I have no desire to drink any more than this.

Moreover, I haven't eaten even a slice of meat for nearly twenty years now. This is not something I deliberately set out to do. After I had spent three months learning Yoga at the holy land of the Himalayas where there was a strict vegetarian diet, I went down the mountain and ordered a curry at a restaurant in New Delhi. The curry that came was mutton curry, and when the smell of meat reached my nose, I realized then that my appetite for it had completely vanished. Before going to the Himalayas I had loved eating meat, but from that time forth I stopped eating it for good.

It is not just me who has had this type of experience. My Yoga students also tell me of similar experiences. I heard from one of my students who practised Yoga continually for some time, that the amount of coffee consumed everyday naturally went down from ten cups to two cups. Another student told me that five bowls of rice were usually needed to become full but after continuing with Yoga, only one bowl was now sufficient.

This is why I do not think it necessary to force any change in your diet. Instead, if you do Yoga, as your body de-stresses it will come to realize it wants good things and will distance itself from bad things. In this way, your diet will naturally become healthy.

Chapter 9: Life And Meditation

Why Should We Do Meditation?

According to the theory of reincarnation, between dying in the previous world and receiving life again in the next, the spirit stays in a middle world. The time spent here is called 'Chū' in Chinese Buddhism and 'Barudo' in Tibetan Buddhism. While in this world the spirit understands everything, and every thought is turned immediately into reality. When the soul is in this middle world, it plans the next life in order to rectify the effects of any bad actions made in the last life. In this middle world where thought immediately turns into reality, there is no effort involved. We are thus born again into the world where we can follow through with the plans made. When we are born here, the memories from our past life have usually been erased, and the plans made by our spirit in the middle world are put into action by the great power of the Universe for us to undertake. We are thus tested to see whether or not we can live this life the way we planned we would live it.

Bearing this in mind, we can say that meditation is for remembering our own divinity and original essential existence as a spirit. Meditation is there for us to realize the truth, which is that we all have a spiritual existence.

In other words, meditation awakens the spirit and is one of the ways of reminding us of the reason why we are living here in this moment.

Through meditation, we can meet our true selves, and understand that everything is one. This personal realization will have a significant effect on how we view the world. From this realization we can become happy and be at peace with ourselves.

When we look back on the day just passed, we realize how much we get caught up in an overflowing whirlpool of thoughts and ideas. From the moment we get up to the time we go to bed at night we think incessantly, unable to put a stop to the constant chattering of the mind.

Because of this incessant inner chatter, we recall what happened in the past, and feel regret, anger, sadness, depression, and anxiety about the future. We then become ill because of the stress. All these many thousands of thoughts and ideas in the mind make us suffer.

From ages past, religion has devised various ways to stop and control these thoughts. In the Yoga Sutras it states, "Yoga stops the movement of the mind."

When we meditate, the mind is fixed on one point and gradually we can feel the chattering of the mind die down. From here the inward journey begins. Soon, in the silence of your heart, you will feel a calming sensation. Peace will then take over your mind.

When you can stop the chattering in the mind for a long duration, you can then start using the intuitive mind that had until this point been dormant. As a result, you will start to understand things better and become wiser.

Soon, with silence of heart, you will become an observer to things without being swayed by them. Through mere observation you will understand the whole picture and will grasp the essential nature of things. You will thus see clearly what is important for you and what is not. Without being misled into believing anything that is distorted on a conscious or subconscious level, you are able to see things as they really are and you will have conviction in whatever you do.

Once our uncertainty disappears, our attachment to things will fade away. We suffer because we have likes and dislikes, and because we are attached to things. When this attachment disappears, feelings of gentleness, of wanting to be fair to all; feelings abound with love will naturally take their place.

The more our shackles disappear, the more we focus on our consciousness and a realization is born deep in the mind. In the Yoga Sutras it teaches how once the chattering of the mind is cut off, a 'true self' appears. It is said that this 'true self' lives an absolutely free, independent existence, unrestricted by time, space and is always overflowing with peace and light.

In this way, as we learn how to deepen our meditation, we begin to realize our spiritual essence of being. We remember that the true self is a timeless spiritual existence.

Once this is realized, a sense of contentment and peace comes from within, bringing a state of mind that cannot be affected or swayed by other people or external things.

The Object Of Concentration Should Be Something You Are Fond Of

In order to do meditation, it is necessary to concentrate on something. Let us look into the method of this spiritual concentration.

There are two ways, depending on the object of concentration. There is the choice of concentrating on things within yourself or on things outside yourself. Incidentally,

The object of concentration can be anything as long as it is not something bad.

The outside objects to concentrate on could include a statue of Buddha, the Mandala (a painting of Buddha) or the flame of a candle. You could also concentrate on something in the natural world such as the evening sun, the stars, a mountain, or the sea. Alternatively you could chant mantras, or read sutras while concentrating on your voice.

The inner things that you could concentrate on include the space between the eyebrows, the tip of the nose, the 'tanden' (the area below the belly button), the heart, or another part of the body. Alternatively, you could concentrate on your own breathing, or on an image of a lotus flower in your mind.

Once you start concentrating on something, distracting thoughts and images will arise one after the other. This is because by concentrating on one thing, your conscious mind fades away, and the thoughts of your unconscious, which had been pushed down, come to the surface. Just observe these thoughts as they spring up, and let them take their course. If you do this, they will gradually die down.

When the concentration of your spirit is going well, your breathing will become extremely slow and rhythmical. This level of concentration of the spirit when it is fixed on a particular thing is called 'Dharana' (concentration) in Yoga.

In the Yoga Sutras, it states that "concentration (or Dharana) is when the mind binds itself to a particular place" (from the Japanese translation by the late Dr. Tsuruji Sahoda).

Dr. Sahoda mentions in his translation that concentration is the opposite of suppressing the external senses. Rather, it is actively and voluntarily choosing a particular place and binding the mind to it, a form of psychological manipulation. Here the word 'place' implies that the subject of the concentration is a specific thing. For example, the end of the nose, a part of the body like the belly button, or an appropriate thing in the outside world can be chosen as a subject to concentrate on. He goes on, "To bind may be quite a direct expression, but it indicates specifically that the mind is in an unmovable, fixed state."

Next, the distracting thoughts from the subconscious disappear when the soul merges with the subject it is concentrating on. This relatively long and continuous spiritual concentration is called Dhyana (meditation) in Yoga. In the Yoga Sutras it states, "meditation follows from concentration, and happens when you merge with what you are concentrating on and keep in this state."

Dr. Sahoda says that meditation (Dhyana) is called 'Zenna' in Buddhism and is the most central process of the psychological manipulations in Yoga. For example if you choose a flower to be the subject, you will lose all interest in everything except the flower, and it will burn with extreme clarity in you mind. Once you succeed in doing this, move your concentration to various things in connection with the flower, developing the thoughts as far as you can in the same level of clarity as before.

Not only the colour of the flower, the shape and the smell, but also where it came from, who gave it to you, and so on and so forth.

"This is a pure consciousness that carries effortlessly on and on", Dr. Sahoda explains. "This is the state of meditation, and it flows on until you reach a state of deep contemplation."

We can tell whether or not we have entered this state of meditation by checking our breathing. If it has stopped naturally, or is in a quiet state where you cannot really tell, and if this carries on for about three to five minutes, then you are in meditation.

Last of all is the final level of spiritual concentration. In Yoga this is called 'Samadhi' (contemplation), the state of enlightenment.

In the Yoga Sutras, it says, "enlightenment happens when you are in a meditative state, and you become the actual object of your thought, as if your body has disappeared." To put it simply, Samadhi happens when the person enters a deeper state of meditation and merges with the thing they are meditating on, so that no differentiation can be made between the two. According to one expert in meditation, when you enter this deep contemplative state, your breathing will all but stop for more than twelve minutes. Normally this would mean you would die, but apparently the reason you do not is because your spirit is governing your physical body.

This type of breathing is called 'fourth level breathing' in the Yoga Sutras.

This is the state of trance (superconsciousness) which is found in both the internal breathing technique of the mystical thinker Swedenborg who claims to have explored the supernatural world, and the abdominal breathing of the Chinese Sendō. The Indian mystic, Paramahansa Yogananda said that "inhalation provides the exhalation and exhalation provides the inhalation" and, explaining what it says in the Yoga Sutras, said "liberation depends on Pranayama (breathing exercises). Pranayama reaches completion when breathing can be brought to a standstill."

In other words, the last stage for spiritual breathing is of deep contemplation, where the breathing is of no breathing.

To help us understand concentration, meditation and deep contemplation we can look at it in the following way.

Firstly, imagine some water in a cup and concentrate on it. Soon, your mind will fix on the water (concentration). When this happens, imagine various things to do with the water. For example, when you drink it, it runs down your throat into the internal organs then leaves the body as urine. This water then joins with rain water and flows down a river until it reaches the sea. In the sea the water is heated up and is evaporated by the sun, becoming a cloud in the sky. It then soon becomes a rain cloud and is rained down upon a forest. It then flows back into a river where it is stopped by a dam. This water is then taken up by the water mains where it becomes drinking water and returns again to being inside a cup. (Meditation).

When you meditate on this kind of thing over and over again, you and the water cease to be separate things; you will become the water. You will then experience what it is like to be the water. You will pass down the throat, go around the internal organs then leave the body. You will then become one with the rain and flow into a river, reaching the sea where you will evaporate into a cloud, soon to be let down again as rain on the earth where you will make your way back into a cup. (Deep contemplation).

If you make an image like this then you may also come to an understanding of what concentration, meditation and deep contemplation is.

There was a very interesting story in a book I once read regarding this state of oneness with the object of meditation.

Mr. Isamu Mochizuki

Once, a young man became the disciple of a famous Yoga practitioner. This Yoga teacher told the young man to do spiritual concentration. However, he couldn't concentrate due to distracting thoughts that kept on filling his mind. When he brought this up with the teacher, he was asked what he was fond of the most.

"I adore the little baby calf I left behind in my village" he replied.

"Well then", the teacher told him, "don't worry about the spiritual concentration, just think about this baby cow you are very fond of, picture it vividly in your mind from its head down to its tail everyday, from morning till night."

A couple of weeks later, the teacher came to see the young man.

"I think that's enough. You can come out of your room now", he said.

"I can't," the young man replied. "My horns are stuck in the doorway."

The young man had pictured vividly in his mind the baby cow that he loved so much everyday, from morning until evening, until finally he actually became the calf itself. This story explains clearly the state of actually becoming the thing you are imagining (Samadhi).

When I read this story, I felt I understood what this man had experienced since I myself have had a similar experience to this.

When I was in my twenties, I had an experience of staying in a Kibbutz in Israel. While I was there, I caught a chameleon and kept it as a pet. I never grew tired from staring at it everyday. One day I was watching an ant crawl near the chameleon. I was looking at this ant closely for a long time when suddenly I became it. To my utter bewilderment the chameleon appeared as a huge dinosaur from prehistoric time. Even though just for a short moment, I had become indistinguishable from the ant.

Speaking from this experience, if you are finding it hard to do spiritual concentration, then choose something close to your heart as an object to meditate on.

It says in the Yoga Sutras that "meditating on something you are fond of will bring about a stillness in the mind." (Translation by Dr. Sahoda).

Dr. Sahoda adds, "this is regardless of what kind of subject it is you choose. As long as it is something you are fond of or has an influence over you, be it an outside object, or an inner one, an abstract thing or something specific, it does not matter. The only condition is that it is not something bad."

Yoga Trains The 'Plant' Nerve (The Mind and The Soul)

I have noticed various things from observing people who have just started practicing Yoga.

The first thing they realize is that they either stop catching colds, or they get over them very quickly. Ill people get healthy, and healthy people get amazingly healthy.

The reason for this is that Yoga stimulates the sympathetic nerve and the parasympathetic nerve of the autonomic nervous system in turns, which strengthens the inside of the body. After doing a pose in Yoga, we must relax. In a pose, the body is bent forward, backward and twisted and this stimulates the sympathetic nerve. Afterwards when we lie down and relax, in order to calm the excited nerve, the parasympathetic nerve starts to work. When this parasympathetic nerve is activated effectively, we become deeply and comfortably relaxed.

The main thing we can wish for from doing Yoga is achieving this deep, blissful relaxation. Therefore, no matter how beautifully we do the pose, if we do not relax then our attempts at doing Yoga are meaningless. Practising Yoga as a stretching exercise or a workout may have aesthetic value but it is missing the fundamental point of Yoga.

Doing Yoga strengthens the source of true power. This source of true power lies in the unseen, discreet part of the body. Since Yoga builds up this unseen source of power, we overcome any illness we have, and become slim and healthy.

On the other hand, doing Sports trains the power of the muscles, but not so much the insides. Maybe it is because of this that from time to time physically muscular athletes catch colds before an important event or are unable to perform well even though they make extra care to prevent this from happening. Rather than do Sports because it makes you healthy, people think it far more important to break records. In reality, there are many people who, by forcing themselves to do this, damage their health.

Yoga is not just about becoming healthy. At the same time your features will also rapidly improve. An ashen grey face will become clear and radiant. The change can go deeper. A gloomy person will become bright and cheerful, a persistent worrier will stop fretting, and a temperamental person will become gentle. In this way, the character of the person will start to become better.

I wonder if there are many people who have improved their character or personality from doing sports.

Why is it that even though both Sports and Yoga train the body they are different in this way?

The studies of Dr. Shigeo Miki, a scholar in autopsy, gave me a hint as to why this is.

Dr. Shigeo Miki (1925-1987) graduated from the faculty of medicine at Tokyo University, moved on to the autopsy department and then again to the autopsy department of the Tokyo Medical and Dental University before becoming a professor (Doctor of medicine) at the Tokyo National University of Fine Arts and Music. He asserts that the mind or soul is not found in the brain, but in the internal organs. I was very surprised by Dr. Miki's ideas, but since I knew of the awareness in the world of fast progressing research on the brain and also possibly because I do Yoga, I could accept them readily.

He says that "human beings consist of a plant-like part and an animal-like part which are merged together." ('The motion of the internal organs and the mind of a child', published by Tsukiji Shokan). In other words, a plant nerve and an animal nerve.

The plant nerve is in the bowels, veins and kidneys, etc, and is called 'the internal organ group', while the animal nerve is in the 'animal organs' such as the muscles, nerves and skin, etc, and is called the 'body-wall group'. Here is an explanation to make it easier to understand. Dr. Miki says "when you cut a fish open and take out its guts, this is the 'internal organ group', and the bit left over which you can eat is called the 'body-wall group'. The head has both parts in it."

This internal organ system of the plant nerve is hardly influenced at all by the body-wall group of the animal nerve. This we can tell clearly from drinking a hot cup of tea. We can feel the hotness of the tea until the throat area, but we stop feeling it when it passes down from there.

Despite this, the animal nerve is influenced by the plant nerve. Say, for example, you have to cancel meeting up with a friend because you have a bad stomach from eating too much the night before. Here the plant nerve of the stomach senses that it is not in great condition and transmits this to the animal nerve of the brain. The brain thinks, "I don't want to go out and meet my friend" and decides to cancel the appointment. It is not *you* who cancelled the appointment because your stomach started acting strange. The sense in your internal organs cancelled it.

In this way, the mind exists in the internal organs. In Japanese there are the sayings such as 'I have a restless worm in my stomach', meaning to be angry, 'my stomach is boiling over', meaning to be livid, 'speak with the stomach wide open', meaning to speak honestly, 'black stomach', meaning sinister, 'stomach acting', meaning to be scheming, 'to search the stomach', meaning to bring out the truth in someone and 'fat belly' meaning someone who remains unfazed. It could be said, therefore, that people long ago made such proverbs as they believed that the mind and true feelings exist in the stomach.

The old sayings are not only associated with the stomach. There are also the expressions, 'a strong heart' and 'hair growing on the heart', both describing a shameless, cocky person. In English, 'to have a broken heart' can be used for someone disappointed in love, and in Japanese, 'the chest is excited' for when we worry about something. People long ago assumed that the mind lived in the heart; I doubt it was just superstition.

Incidentally, in America, since the introduction of organ transplants, a strange thing started to happen. It is said that the patients who received a heart or lung transplant adopted the mind of the organ donors. Apparently, notes of these experiences by the recipients of organ transplants are published in America.

In the book, 'The mind is a product of the internal organs' (Japan Broadcast Publishing Co., Ltd.), Dr. Katsunari Nishihara, a doctor of medicine who was present at some of the lectures of Dr. Shigeo Miki about the study of life forms in the field of autopsy states that "the most important thing to recognize is that even if you transplant the brain of a shark into a rat, or the brain cells of a foetus into an adult human being, the cells only serve as a transistor, through which an electric current is distributed. From this we can gather that even if brain cells are transplanted, no change will occur in the mind. On the other hand, the fact that in organ transplants the mind also changes tells us that the whereabouts of the mind is in the internal organs." He states that from the preferences of colour to likes and dislikes of food, all is governed by the internal organs.

Dr. Shigeo Miki goes on to express his thought on the relationship between the head and the mind.

When we express the Kanji character of the Japanese word for 'to think', 思 'omoi', hieroglyphically it is said that the pattern shows the head 頭 'atama', lending an ear to the mind or soul, 心 'kokoro'. The origin of the upper part 田 of the character 思 is ▨, which shows the brain from a birds eye view. The lower part 心 of 思 is from the hieroglyph ⌇, which is a heart. 思 is therefore a composition which very clearly shows how the plant nerve supports the animal nerve. ('Jitsū' by Prof. Shizuka Shirakawa, published by Heibonsha Limited, Tokyo).

He goes on from this to outline the differences between thinking with the heart and with the mind.

Just like the statue of Miroku Bosatsu (the Buddha of the future) in Koryuji (a famous temple in Kyoto, Japan), a person who thinks with the heart is one who has a straight back, and who listens to his own plant-like inner nature, quietly vibrating in resonance with the Cosmos.

The person who thinks with the head is on the other polar extreme. An example of this is Rodin's 'the Thinker'. The mouth is covered, and the body is bent over as if to shut off the plant nerve. It is a pose where the animalist extremes of sense, feeling and action are pushed out to the fore, and where the brain is hard at work, thinking.

Dr. Shigeo Miki's ideas really compounded my own belief that Yoga trains the inner organs and the plant nerve, developing and elevating the mind and soul.

In Sports, no matter how much you train the body, the mind and soul will remain unchanged. Granted, training the body will develop the body and the senses. Martial Arts, for instance, train the animal nerve the most by building the body up and sharpening the senses to the extreme. If, however, from all the hard work and perseverance a person reaches the peak of his sport and becomes world champion, while it may be something to be admired, can it be said that in doing so, they have acquired a great personality and wonderful humanity? I do not think that by merely training the animal nerve, a person can improve his character. The important thing is to train the plant nerve.

In recent years, Computer Games and the Internet have become very popular with young people. When we think about it, their animal nerves are in overdrive since they are constantly using their fingertips and brains. I think that it is possibly this extreme imbalance between the animal and the plant nerve that is responsible for desensitizing the minds of people nowadays.

Although man's sense of the world around him has developed through the ages, there is a part that has remained unchanged for thousands of years; the plant nerve of the internal organs. If you read 'The Tale of Genji', for instance, a novel written a thousand years ago, what strikes you is how little the mind of the human being has changed since then.

It is especially necessary for us now to train the plant nerve and control the unruly animal nerve. In so doing we can develop and improve the soul. One method that makes this possible is Yoga.

Chapter 10: The Power Of Life. Methods Of Practice.

A Method To Prevent Oneself From Slipping Into Despair

Words of comfort or encouragement are of no use to those who, because they cannot face the onset of old age, illness, and death, are on the brink of despair. People like this need a precise set of points of advice. Here are some points they can work on.

The first point is to make sure that what you take in through your eyes is imprinted, from moment to moment, on your mind.

It is said that when most people get old, they enter a circle of depression where all they can think of is imminent immobility, illness and death. Even thinking of death in a metaphysical way does not bring any relief.

Let me show you a method based on my own experience as described in the section 'Place your mind in the moment and things will become easy'. (Chapter Two)

From each moment to the next, take in everything you feel, such as the emotions of joy, sadness, the appreciation of beauty and the sense of gratitude and imprint these feelings on the mind. As you do this, the time you live will become full and rich, and at the end of every day you will be satisfied that you have had an enjoyable day. Experiencing this will liberate you from constantly thinking of death and despair.

The second point is to believe that for yourself, there is no death.

Once in the middle of my travels as a youth there was a period of time when I was haunted by the fear of death. I was around the River Ganges in India, and saw an old man waiting for death to take him when a message appeared in my mind; "death does not exist until we die." At that moment my mind immediately felt at ease.

What I had gained from this experience was the knowledge that since we cannot experience our own death, for us there is no death. When I realized this I was liberated from my fear of dying. The thought 'for me there is no death' gives us the power to escape from the fear of dying.

The third point is to change your point of view and hold an unshakable faith.

Say we go down with an incurable illness and fall into despair- what would be the best way to live our life?

If we cannot change our surroundings or our physical body, the only thing we can do is to change how we look at things.

There is a person who completely changed how he saw the world and so managed to live through a time of despair. He is the psychologist Dr. Viktor E. Frankl, a survivor of Auschwitz.

In the concentration camps, where people were sent to their deaths in the gas chambers, where there was hard labour and where typhoid infections were rife, Frankl lived with the fear of not knowing when death would come knocking on his door.

In these conditions, he gave up any expectations he had and instead attributed a special meaning to the events that happened in his life. To live includes suffering and dying. Although his destiny may have been to have a life of suffering, everything that happens is only for this moment, and will never happen again. When he reached this understanding, he was delivered from his anxiety.

In his book, 'Ein Psychologe Erlebt Das Konzentrationslager' (literal translation: 'A Psychologist Experiences The Concentration Camp'; English title: Man's Search for Meaning) he writes of how, just from thinking this thought, he was able to stand firm in the midst of despair.

As well as changing how we view the world, we must also have an unshakable faith. Wandering alone in the desert on my travels, I experienced first hand just how much life force can be generated from having an unwavering belief.

There is no need for God or religion. If you hold an unshakeable belief and fill every nook and cranny of your inner self with it, you will receive the power to rise up from the brink of despair.

The Method Of Meditation From The Desert

In my youth, I devised and practiced a 'desert meditation method' from my wanderings in the desert. Here is part of the method, called 'desert image training' which is a way of getting rid of unwanted thoughts in the mind.

The first thing to do is to sit or lie down in a quiet room and relax. Now picture the desert in your mind. The blue sky and sand expands out before you. In this desert you are walking alone.

When any unwanted thoughts rise up in your mind, imagine picking them up one by one with your hands and throwing them away. Since you are walking in the desert, they fall down behind you and soon disappear.

If, after a while, unwanted thoughts still rise up in your mind, keep picking them up and throwing them behind you.

It is important to picture yourself walking. When you walk you get further and further away from the thoughts you have discarded which soon disappear. Until you are at peace, keep walking and throwing away the unwanted thoughts.

Now, just as the ground is singed and purified by the scorching sun of the desert, so are your unpleasant thoughts and the things that hold you back in your life. When you finish this, imagine coming to an oasis in the desert, and rest comfortably in the shade of a tree until you are satisfied.

I am sure that if you can clearly imagine the blue sky, the sweeping sand of the desert, walking alone in the desert, the burning sun and the shade under the tree in the oasis, you will be able to liberate yourself from unwanted thoughts and become at peace with yourself.

The Method For Sharpening Your Powers Of Intuition

Intuition is when, in a blink of an eye, you understand everything without the use of thought. Intuition is like the wisdom of 'satori' (enlightenment) and happens when you access the answers of the Universe, which have been there all along.

In order to sharpen your powers of intuition concerning a particular problem, you should firstly be mindful of the problem at hand, and then relax. At the same time, you should look within yourself and be sensitive of your own feelings as you go about your daily life.

For example, consider a specific problem. If you have no clue as to how to solve it, look within yourself and be sensitive of your own feelings as you go about your daily life. If you pass your days like this, there is a chance the answer will suddenly come up from within yourself and make itself known to you. It may also come out unexpectedly from watching the TV, reading the newspaper or a magazine, or from a conversation with a friend.

If you are not sensitive enough, you will miss these signs from your intuition. However, if you relax, and go about your daily life alert and mindful of your inner state of mind then your powers of intuition will most certainly increase.

A Method For Boosting Your Level Of Ki

The first condition for boosting your level of Ki is to be able to relax deeply.

Ki works on both mind and matter, so if you cannot relax or are not in the mood then it will not come out. If you don't feel like doing the Ki exercises therefore, you should not force yourself.

The same goes for breathing exercises. There are a lot of breathing exercises, more than one might expect. I myself know around sixty. If it is a pleasant feeling of relaxation you want from a breathing exercise I would say any one of the following will do.

An important thing to remember is to be both relaxed and have an appropriate amount of tension in the body. A straight back is important since it means a bit of tension remains while you are relaxed. It is possible to do it lying down, but in this case there is no tension, and one normally ends up going to sleep. When this happens no Ki can come out.

Let's have a go at sensing Ki. First, sit with your back straight. Now, concentrating on your breath, slowly exhale the air in your lungs. It is important when doing this to put your mind into your exhalation. Now exhale further, drawing your stomach in as you do so. When you have exhaled all you can, just relax, and you should inhale automatically. The amount of air that you had exhaled will be inhaled naturally. Once you have repeated this several times, bring the palms of your hands together. You should be able to feel a slight tingling or a warm ball of energy.

I recommend you try lots of different breathing exercises to see which ones suit you best then practise these on a daily basis. A simple breathing exercise which you can do comfortably and for long is the one to do.

A Breathing Exercise For People Who Find It Hard To Sleep At Night

For those who cannot sleep at night, have a tired head, or who become tense and find it hard to relax while flying, there is a particular breathing method I would like to recommend; the breathing exercise for the brain. I found this method in the book 'Nō kokyū' ('Brain Breathing' by Seung Heung Lee and others, published by Business Sha Publishers). I tried it out and am convinced of its benefits.

It is a simple technique, but since the 'tsubo' (pressure points) on the head are used, it is necessary to memorize where the points are. If you memorize these 'tsubo' and use them for breathing you will, I am sure, be surprised at how effective it is. If you do this exercise just twice in succession, your head will feel as light as a feather and you will be able to relax.

Please look at the diagram on page 168.

To begin with, as you breathe in, imagine you are bringing in your breath slowly from the tsubo at the crown of your head (1- Hyakue). Now, very slowly breathe out from your mouth. As you breathe out, imagine that all the stagnant and negative energy is being released from your body.

Now breathe through the other tsubo in the following order.

2- Zenchō (about five centimetres in front of the Hyakue tsubo).

3- Indō (the centre of the forehead)

4- Miken (in between the eyebrows)

5- Taiyō (both temples).

6- Jinchū (under the nose).

7- Amon (between the second and third vertebrae from the top of the neck).

8- Gyokuchin (the two bits below the two lumps at the base of the head).

As you repeat this exercise, you will get the feeling that your breath is a thin stream coming into your brain from each tsubo.

Mr. Isamu Mochizuki

I recommended this technique to people suffering from insomnia and they told me that since they had started practicing it they were able to sleep without using sleeping pills and were much more awake in the morning.

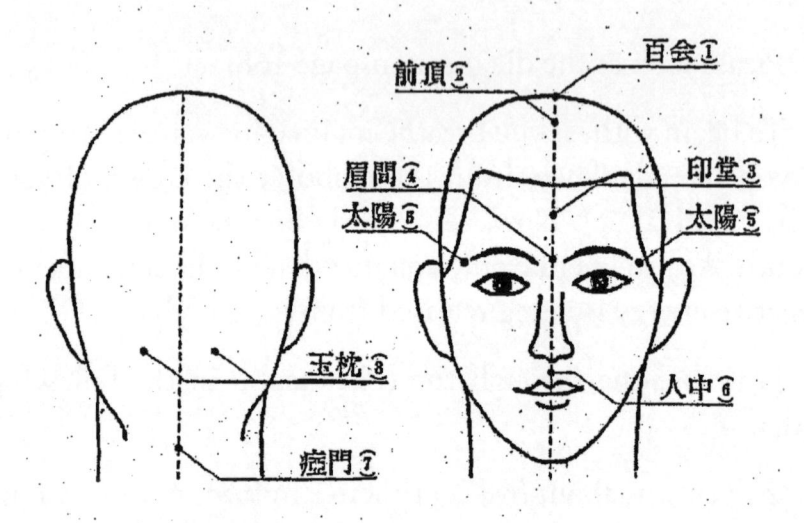

1- Hyakue

2- Zenchō

3- Indō

4- Miken

5- Taiyō

6- Jinchū

7- Amon

8- Gyokuchin

A Method For Receiving The Energy Of The Sun Into The Body When You Get Up In The Morning

I recommend the 'Sun worship' pose to feel fresh and invigorated in the morning when getting up. However, since there are twelve movements to do for this pose, it is difficult and a bother for those just starting out.

I have therefore devised a pose with just three movements which are easy to remember and hardly take any time to do.

The pose goes in the following order.

1- In the morning, face the sun (if you cannot see the sun from where you are, picture it in your mind), stand with your legs together and put your hands together in front of your chest as if to pray.

2- While breathing in slowly, raise your arms and stretch backwards. When breathing in, imagine the energy of the sun filling your body.

3- Now breathe out, bending the top half of your body right down until your fingertips touch the floor. When they do, you should have exhaled out all that you can. As you breathe out, imagine that all the stagnant and negative energy is being released from your body.

4- Breathe in slowly, while returning to the pose in (1).

Repeat 1 to 4 two times. To finish, lie down and relax.

Once I watched a program on TV which compared the brain activity in the morning for people who had slept on a bed to people who had slept on a futon. There was seen to be an increase in brain activity just from the action of picking up and putting the futon away in the closet.

Therefore, if you just do the three basic movements listed above, you will definitely start to feel more fresh and invigorated in the morning. Once you get used to practicing it regularly, it might then be an idea to have a go at the full Sun worship pose.

A Pose You Can Do For A Good Night's Sleep

Before bedtime, the best Yoga pose to do is the one where you bend your body forwards. Try it and you will become relaxed and your anxieties will disappear.

The poses where you bend backwards work in the opposite way, stimulating your spine and making your head feel sharp and alert.

Try the pose where you bend forwards in the following way:

1- Put your feet together and sit with your legs stretched out in front of you.

2- Now clasp your toes. Those who cannot reach their toes, hold your ankles.

3- While breathing out slowly, draw your stomach in and curve your back.

4- Now as you slowly breathe in, raise the top half of your body and look at the ceiling.

5- As you slowly breathe out, bend the top half of your body as far down as you can. Hold your breath at this point.

6- Finally, as you breathe in slowly, raise your top half of your body again, back to the original position.

Repeat this process again, but the second time at (4), when you bend your top half forwards, stay in this position and breathe normally for ten to twenty seconds.

You can now get into your bed, but before going to sleep, cleanse your mind. To cleanse your mind, picture something beautiful that you have seen, such as a clear running stream or a snow-capped mountain range. Just by remembering such beautiful scenes your mind will be influenced at a deep level of your subconsciousness. You will now be able to sleep soundly.

The Way To Use Ki When You Want To Make Your Point Known To Someone

When we look at the natural world, we can see that there is always a positive and negative side to everything, something I touched on in Chapter Five. Even an egg or a plant has positive and negative sides, a fact you can prove with a voltmeter.

In the same way, the earth too has a North pointing pole and a South pointing pole.

Just like this, our bodies too have polarity. The right side of the body is positive and the left side is negative. Also, the top half of the body is positive and the bottom, negative.

Ki comes out from the positive side and comes in from the negative side. For the arms, the Ki comes out of the right hand and into the left hand. For the eyes, Ki exits the right eye and enters the left eye.

Once you know about the polarity of the body, it is possible to apply this knowledge to practical use.

For example, when you are desperate to make someone understand your intentions, you should sit on their left, and stare with your right eye at the left eye or the left side of the person while you make your case. Before you know it, the person will start to come round to your point of view and agree with you even though you may not understand how or why.

The reason this happens can be thought of in the following way. The left eye is connected to the right side of the brain, and the right eye is connected to the left side of the brain. Therefore it may be that when you concentrate on the left eye of a person, the waveforms generated from your will are directly channeled into the right side of their brain (the imagination side), and this, combined with Ki makes it easy for them to agree with you.

An Easy Way To Relax While Lying Down

If you can do hypnosis well on yourself, you will be able to relax deeply just by lying down. I talked about this in Chapter Two, but let us go over it again.

To be hypnotized by someone can sometimes be dangerous, but if you are just doing it to yourself it is perfectly safe.

Firstly, lie down and think to yourself, "the toes on my right foot are now relaxed."

Now do the same to your right ankle, right calf, right knee and right thigh. Repeat this with the left leg.

Next, the large intestine, the stomach, the heart, the lungs and the neck. After this, the right hand finger tips, the right wrist, right elbow and right shoulder.

Repeat this for the left arm. Now continue up with the chin, mouth, nose, ears, eyes, forehead and the top of the head.

Now think to yourself "my arms have become heavy." Imagine both arms are comfortably and firmly stuck to the floor. Then imagine that your back is comfortably stuck firm to the floor. Now imagine your legs have become heavy and are stuck firmly to the floor.

Finally, imagine that your whole body is comfortably attached to the floor. Your body and mind are now perfectly relaxed.

After practicing this for a while, you will get the knack of releasing the tension in the body, and may start dropping off to a comfortable sleep even before you get to the stomach area.

An Exceptionally Easy Way To Get Rid Of The Ailments Of The Body

In Yoga, there are a number of methods for getting rid of illnesses in the body.

They require you, however, to memorize various Yoga poses. For those who find this a bother to do, I recommend the following ultra-easy method.

Long ago there lived a French psychotherapist named Émile Coué (1857-1926) who invented this method, called 'The Coué Method'.

It is unbelievably simple to do.

Repeat to yourself, "Day by day, in every way, I am getting better and better." That's all there is to it.

Many people suffering from serious diseases have got better from doing this method. I too have recommended it to various people suffering from ill health, and it does indeed seem to work.

Repeat these words parrot-like to yourself, day in, day out, to really lodge them in the brain. If you do this, you will be surprised to see a daily improvement in your health.

Afterword

I am sure that when anyone looks back on their life, they will see a number of turning points. One of the turning points in my life was when I quit my job after three years as a businessman and decided to go abroad.

When I quit the company I was working for, lots of people around me tried to stop me. My job was going well, and my company had some faith in me. There seemed no reason to quit.

However, no matter how hard I tried, I could not get rid of my feelings of discontentment. "Twenty-five, and no job. What on earth are you going to do?" echoed the various voices of criticism around me. In spite of this, I decided to go abroad.

Only my mother remained unopposed to such a self-centred decision. "If there is something you want to do, you must try it," she said.

I therefore quit my job, and set out on my travels overseas. First, I went to London where I worked part-time and studied at a language school. After that I stayed in Madrid and travelled around Europe before moving on to Israel and becoming a volunteer in a Kibbutz.

After wandering the Shinai peninsula, I went to Sweden to earn some money for travelling, then traversed the land from Europe to India. From here I went to Nepal and on to Sri Lanka, before finally returning home to Japan after a five-year hiatus.

During my travels, I descended into a pit of anxiety and self-loathing because I did not know what on earth I was doing. I still had not discovered the thing I wanted to do.

Driven by my anxiety, I made my way back to London, passing through Morocco, Algeria and the expanse of the Sahara desert. I then went to Tanzania in East Africa and from there on to Kenya, Ethiopia, and Egypt. In these travels, many nights were spent sleeping rough.

From there I crossed over to Jordan, then passed through Syria, Turkey and Greece, before arriving back in London. It had been a seven month long trip.

When I was staying at a cheap inn in Africa, I learnt a little Shōrinji Kempō (a Martial Art) from a university student. When I got back to England, I immediately got in contact with the British Shōrinji Kempō Federation and started training. I carried this on for as long as ten years.

During this time I also tried Yoga, Ki therapy, Chinese martial arts and breathing exercises amongst other things.

From starting Yoga in particular, I was able to look into myself and discover what I had been searching for all along. This surprised me greatly.

I realized that I had taken the long way round, just like the boy in the story 'The Blue Bird' by Maeterlinck, who sets out on his travels to search for the blue bird only to return home empty handed and find that it had been there all along.

However, when I look back on it now I realize that taking the long way round had not been a waste of time. Rather it had been a valuable experience. After all, in life there is no such thing as a worthless experience.

In Shōrinji Kempō there is a method called 'Seihō'. It is a method used for fixing dislocations or for returning a person back to consciousness after a blackout.

In the Dōjō (training hall), when someone damaged a joint I would sometimes be the one to apply 'Seihō' on them. There were times when I hadn't even put my hand on the person when they would say to me "the pain has gone." Since I hadn't actually done anything I thought this very odd. As this continued to happen I began to realize that a force, separate from the method I was using, was at work.

To add to this, a funny thing happened when I started practicing Yoga by myself. I was in a pose where I was standing on one leg, and when I raised my hands (together as if for prayer) above my head while breathing in, something hot shot up from my feet to the top of my head and my hands started to tingle. When I stretched out my palms, to put it rather dramatically, it felt as if they were being charged with an electric current.

Also, when I did Yoga poses where the body is twisted, I started to notice a fragrant aroma given off.

I became convinced that this was the work of Ki. I was truly amazed by the power of Yoga.

I talked about this to some English Yoga veterans who had been practicing for ten or twenty years. They told me that they had never had such an experience. Since I had thought that everyone doing Yoga experienced this, I wondered what on earth it could be.

I then realized that this was 'Prana' in Yoga, or 'Ki'.

After I realized this, I started to collect and emit Ki from my palms and fingertips. As I became able to do this, I also became able to detect the whereabouts of any Ki blockages in the body. When I put Ki into these places I got an immediate response. The flow of Ki became smooth and constant and the symptoms of the illness disappeared.

At that time, I was a businessman in London. As my understanding of Ki deepened, I became more and more unhappy with my job. It finally came to the point where I had to start looking for other work.

Everyday, whilst doing Yoga, I prayed to myself, saying "Please give me a job most suited to me." While I continued to pray I grew more and more certain that there was nothing for me to do other than heal people with Ki. Even though I knew this inside, I still didn't know for sure whether I would be able to earn a living from it.

However, in the midst of my anxiety, I remembered reading about the research the psychologist Dr. Carl Jung had done on fortune telling. He believed that there is a 'synchronicity' (a meaningful coincidence) between the psychological state of the recipient and the advice received.

I therefore approached fortune telling with the belief that it could be used as a type of 'software' to directly listen in to the Universe.

At once I set up a fortune telling kit and used it to ask whether I could become a Ki therapist or not. The advice card that I received was 'The Grace of God'. It read "you are under the blessing of a Great entity." These words resonated to the bottom of my soul.

I decided to quit my job as a businessman. Spurred on by these words of the divination, I proceeded to take my first steps as a Ki therapist.

In the beginning, when people asked me to explain Ki therapy, they would find my answer a little hard to fathom. They would say, "If you could cure illnesses with Ki, there would be no need for doctors."

However, as the amount of people who came to my practice and were healed steadily increased, things spread by word of mouth.

As I started to use Ki on many different people, my perception of health and illness started to change.

Now I think of illness as the proof that we are living, and I think of health as something our consciousness creates. That is why I think that whether you are ill or not, if you believe that you are healthy, then you are healthy. As I began to think in this way, my ideal of how I should live changed. I have put these thoughts of mine into a poem.

I Live By Joining The Flow Of The Universe

My life is just an expanding process.

That is all it is. An expanding process with the Universe.

Simply flowing on, like the flow of time, the flow of a river.

It is not an existence that stops the flow by feeling anger, despair, pride or attachment with things.

Throughout this day, in life's flow, I will do everything that needs to be done.

Get up in the morning, wash my face, do Yoga, meditate.

Eat breakfast, practise Ki therapy, teach Yoga.

I may also travel, meet people, read, write, think, and soak in the bathtub before going to bed.

By doing so I join the flow.

The moment I released myself to the flow, I started to become the flow itself and I gradually felt a change coming over me. Before long, the flow and I became the same thing. By doing Yoga and meditation, all sense of ego vanished from my mind.

Since making a natural transition to a simple diet I stopped praising the virtue of poverty.

By healing other people, I was being healed myself. Through this understanding, any self-pride that I had in doing Ki therapy disappeared.

As I started to teach Yoga, I stopped feeling the need to tell people what to do.

As these changes came about me, I found the flow racing alongside me, or penetrating right through me. And on each day, the good things, the bad things, the serious things, the less serious things, the truth and the untruth that cropped up all became part of the unceasing flow, flowing on and flowing by.

Immersing myself in the main current of the flow, we flow together.

I will not cling on to anything that comes my way, however desirable it may be.

Without any preference to any thing, I can live encompassing every thing.

This is to dissolve into the flow while being conscious of my own existence.

As my true self, to keep on existing in the flow. That is my only role of living.

This book is a collection of my talks at my London Yoga and Ki class which have arisen naturally from a state of deep relaxation with my students.

Even if it is just one part, I would be extremely happy if you can empathise with, put into practice or make use out of anything written in this book for your everyday life.

To end with, I would like to give my heartfelt thanks to Ms.Yūko Ando and Mrs. Fumiyo Watanabe of Yūyū projects, Ms. Kuni Kobashi of Office One, Mr. Jun Mimura who designed the cover and Mr.Takashi Takaoka of Heibonsha Publishers who edited this book.

1st October 2004 at home in London.

Isamu Mochizuki.

Author

Isamu Mochizuki

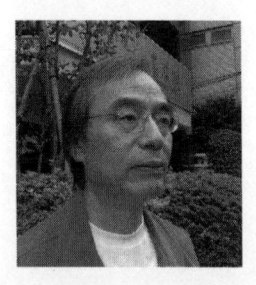

Isamu Mochizuki was born in Japan in 1948. In 1973 at the age of 25, he travelled to London.

After roaming various countries in Europe, he joined a Kibbutz in Israel, and journeyed to the Shinai Peninsula. He then made his way on land through Greece, the Middle East, Turkey, Iran and Afganistan to India and Nepal. He fell ill with acute hepatitis in India and returned back home to Japan.

In 1979 he went back to London. The next year, he travelled on land to Africa. In seven months, he traversed the Sahara desert by hitchhiking and camping outside. Whilst travelling in various countries in Africa, he started to believe in intuition and learnt how to follow it in his daily life.

In 1980, he started learning 'Shōrinji Kempō' and also started to practice Yoga and Ki therapy on his own. As a consequence, his eyes were opened to the world of 'Ki'. In 1986, while in Africa, he discovered he had the ability to heal others. The next year in 1987, he went on a pilgrimage to India, and visited various Yoga practices.

Since then he has set up his own Yoga and Ki therapy practice in London which serves as his base.

Printed in Great Britain
by Amazon